JAMES W. RAMAGE, M.S.W., Ph.D.
Psychotherapist

Author of -
Creating Therapeutic Activity Plans
in Long Term Care Facilities: The Basic Principles

Presents

A CAREGIVER'S TRAINING MANUAL FOR THE ELDERLY: ALZHEIMER'S - OTHER DEMENTIA

A guide to bridging treatment strategies

Improve — maintain activities of daily living
Detailed individualized model teaching plans
Examples of training procedures
Improved teaching techniques

"Reaching in and reaching out to your loved ones
at home or in their living environment."

authorHOUSE®

AuthorHouse™
1663 Liberty Drive, Suite 200
Bloomington, IN 47403
www.authorhouse.com
Phone: 1-800-839-8640

First published by AuthorHouse 6/22/2009

ISBN: 978-1-4389-2366-6 (sc)

Printed in the United States of America
Bloomington, Indiana

This book is printed on acid-free paper.

DISCLAIMER

The author does not directly or indirectly dispense medical advice nor does he use behavioral programming as a form of treatment for inappropriate or maladaptive behavior without medical approval. It is not the intent of the author to diagnose or prescribe. The intent of the author is only to offer behavioral information to assist individuals, families, professionals, health care providers and others in their quest to improve a relative or patients quality of life. The information and solutions offered in this book are intended to serve as guidelines for managing behavior. It is an educational procedure and when used the publisher and author assume no responsibility.

MEMORIAL

In memory of my professional colleagues Dr. Joe D. Woddail, Psychiatrist; Dr. Kenneth Crawford, Chaplain; Dr. David Pittman Johnson, University Professor; and Mr. Milton R. Davis, Licensed Professional Counselor; who prior to their untimely deaths, practiced their professions with vision and compassion. Each communicated their expertise and insight to their patients with whom they labored with gratitude, love and care. Their work was one of divine art of healing which occupied their thinking that one's soul should be healed as well as their physical bodies. To them life was love eternal and immortal – death only a horizon of a higher level of consciousness. They are and will continue to be missed.

James W. Ramage, Ph.D.

DEDICATION

This book is dedicated to the numerous families with whom I have worked over the years developing therapeutic programming, interventions and strategies for the elderly and family members trying to cope with Alzheimer's disease. It is these dedicated men and women who serve as caregivers that I extend my appreciation. I have great respect and admiration for their services as they struggle daily to improve the state of over-all well being of a father, mother, significant family member or to someone they hardly know who is suffering from a condition which they do not fully understand or comprehend. It is to these individuals that I share the following thoughts.

There is no human experience more devastating than the distress caused by Alzheimer's dementia; a progressive, irreversible disease of the brain among the elderly. Such an illness can incapacitate a person, and family members alike. It can damage an individual's principles, commitments, and values. It often produces inappropriate social relationships, and behaviors. It generates discomfort and pain which results in a continual loss of self-esteem and dignity. It forces an individual to live a life with debilitating uncertainties.

On a more personal level this dreaded disease can be likened to some evil trick of nature that preys upon the brain rendering it sick, fractured, and useless. It inhibits the psyche and like drug addiction has strong linkage to depression. It tends to remind one of a diabolical discomfort of being imprisoned in a dark, overheated room, a lonely place where there are no doors or windows. A place where there is no breeze to cool oneself, or a means of escaping from the smothering confinement. It is a place where one is secluded from society, a captive of oneself where they are alone in a dungeon surrounded by darkness, locked away from the human species which represents a spectacular manifestation of life.

Missing from their lives are those human traits of joy, language, love, affection, desire, hope, pride and honor which separates the human being from other living creatures which makes life meaningful. And, then anhedonia creeps in and finally claims the person who once laughed, and cried with us, hugged and loved us only to see their points of life, dim, flicker, fade and eventually go out one, by one, by one....

James W. Ramage, Ph.D.

ACKNOWLEDGEMENTS

The author gratefully acknowledges an intellectual debt of gratitude to B. F. Skinner and more specifically to his volume, science and human behavior, (1953) on operant conditioning. And to the many behaviorists with whom I have worked and studied I extend a special word of appreciation. Also, heartfelt thanks is extended to those unselfish healthcare providers, especially to those seasoned mental health professionals, educators and caregivers who taught me most, if not all, of what I know about behavior. To them I express my thanks for tolerating me. They taught me more than they will ever know.

And as a behavioral practitioner in the field of gerontology I would like to take this opportunity to quickly acknowledge that as a Clinician, I have been greatly influenced and my life enriched by my professional association with the elderly and their families. Their wisdom and perspective, both individually and collectively, on life has been both helpful and beneficial to me. It is with great humility that the author tries to capture throughout this book much of their concerns, strengths and needs as well as their kind and meaningful words -- I value their input.

An appreciation is also extended to the governing Board and Administration of Bibb County Hospital and Nursing home complex in Centreville, Alabama, for their support and dedication to this project. And more specifically special thanks is given to Mr. Terry Smith, CEO of the Facility, for his leadership in constructing a state of the art Nursing Home Complex coupled with a philosophy dedicated to providing a well balanced, well integrated, diversified and comprehensive program of services for the elderly and their families in the community.

The author is particularly grateful to the administrator of the facility, Ms. Kandace Shoults for her enthusiastic, appropriate and timely comments. Her input is valued since she is an innovative nurse practitioner who is dedicated to the team concept and continuity of care in the delivery of services to the elderly. Also, a special appreciation is extended to my colleagues Dr. Lata Patil, Medical Director; Julie Darden, R.N., Director of Nursing; Kenya Parker, B.S.W. and Leslie Kornegay, Social Services; and Florence Elam and Inos Perry, Therapeutic Activities; for their contributions. Their words of wisdom and comments were appreciated. And finally to my daughter, Elizabeth (Beth) Snider, who worked tirelessly editing, and to my wife, Margaret, who proofed and provided timely comments of the material, I am grateful. Without their assistance, and the support of my family, this project could not have been completed.

JOURNEY

April showers, rainbows, earthly splendor, a young man's treat
The path to and from the field worn bare by his feet
Footprints of a husband working his fields, feeling complete
His soul buried in Mother Earth, his love rooted deep in Southern Soil
Through life he battles the elements – the sun, wind and rain, he toils.

Each day at dusk he walks slowly from the field
Tired, hungry, and weary from a hard days work
With bruised knuckles, calloused hands, and weather-beaten face
Worn-out shoes, faded overalls and blue denim shirt
Sun-burned face, wrinkled leather skin – things he can't erase.

A quite and gentle man with an endless love for the sod
Plants that bloom, evening rain, smell of new mowed hay all have a niche
Like Heaven on earth made for man by God
He works his fields – at times penniless but yet rich
Fields of cotton and corn - cows with calves marks his success.

At dark, he walks towards home, a smile on his face, a bounce in his feet
Hurrying at days end to his partner, friend, lover, and wife to meet
A helpmate always standing by the fence waiting to greet
Her husband, a hoe on his shoulder and wild flowers in his hand
An act that only life-long lovers can understand.

Then one evening when they met at the end of the day
The things she loved about him had disappeared – gone away
Unable to speak, his face a dull expression, confused, lost like a child
As a wife of faith, sacrifice, love and care with a desire to please
In horror, she realized she had lost her husband to Alzheimer's Disease.

A caregiver, widow, unexpectedly; lifelong secrets to be later resurrected
Never alone – memories abound. Loving thoughts will comfort she knows
Memories always present like roses planted her spouse found easy to grow
Though caregiving was long, hard, bringing to life storms and strife
A wife thinks of her lost love, giving Thanks to God – for it was life-------

James W. Ramage, Ph.D.

TABLE OF CONTENTS

INTRODUCTION

Care of the elderly presents one of the greatest challenges facing healthcare providers in today's society. The growing population of individuals aged sixty five and over suggests that the challenge will continue well into the twenty first century. Disorders in which clinical deficits in cognition of memory exist, representing a significant change from previous levels of functioning, in the elderly. These disorders constitute a large and growing public health problem with Alzheimer's disease being the most common cause of dementia, a major form of mental impairment in the elderly is a challenge to the Medical and Professional Community. Statistics reveal that five percent or more of this population reside in the nation's nursing homes and long term care facilities. Since a large and growing number of the elderly suffer from various stages of Alzheimer's dementia and the numerous behavior problems associated with the disease nursing home staff should be knowledgeable of the basic principles and techniques of behavior management.

Government estimates suggest that up to four million Americans suffer from severe dementia and an additional one to five million have mild to moderate dementia. Ten times as many people are affected now as they were at the turn of the century, and the number of people with severe dementia is expected to increase significantly. Unless cures, or a means of prevention is found for the common causes of dementia, seven million four hundred thousand Americans will be effected by the year of 2040. This proliferation is not the result of an "epidemic" but rather because more people now survive into the high-risk period for dementia, which is middle age and beyond.

Also, as cognitive functioning declines in this population, skills in activities of daily living in such vital areas as toileting, grooming, dressing, dining are lost. In addition, there will be those individuals with serious overlapping psychiatric problems who have suffered from a mental illness most of their lives and who may or may not have dementia. All these issues which are addressed with other groups exist here and treatment must be provided.

These individuals are often manipulative, frightened, have poor impulse control and suffer from depression -- wherever their illness has taken them in life. One of the most disturbing responses to the aging process is those individuals who often exhibit inappropriate behavior. It is these types of behavior that family members, friends and the public in general cannot readily accept which frequently results in nursing home placement. As this population ages and lives longer more and more of the elderly who are confused and demented will need care that can only be provided in skilled nursing home facilities equipped to provide special care.

These statistics are overwhelming and underscores the immediate urgency for our political, professional, and educational systems to commit themselves to providing the same kind of rigorous problem solving, strategic research, and planning that other behavioral problems have received in our society. Healthcare providers who work with the elderly need specialized training in providing effective behavioral programming for the elderly, their families and to others who provide services to this population. The schools, colleges, universities, and professional organizations can be of particular assistance by offering curriculums in eldercare and providing relevant training materials.

Society must consider the welfare of this growing population of demented elderly citizens. And as healthcare providers we must remember that the care of our elderly residents is an ongoing challenge that needs our critical attention, creative planning and solutions.

The material in this book is an attempt to provide teachers, parents, relatives, immediate family members, and more specifically nursing home personnel with guidelines and approaches which allow them to develop safe, practical and yet effective behavior programs for the elderly. This information is designed to provide the reader with a practical, detailed, but easy to follow blueprint for designing and implementing effective therapeutic environments in nursing homes and long term facilities. It encourages development of a milieu that permits straightforward treatment programming, interventions and strategies to deal effectively with skill loss and maladaptive behavior. Such a therapeutic environment addresses in a psycho-educational manner skill loss in the most basic, essential, and frequently overlooked human behaviors of daily living, which is so essential and necessary in their day to day functioning. Therefore, this book is concerned with the operant conditioning approach to establishing therapeutic environments for the elderly residing in our nursing homes and extended care facilities. More specifically, it addresses those elderly residents in our population suffering from Alzheimer's dementia who have experienced severe skill loss and as a result who are exhibiting maladaptive behavior.

Today, operant behavior modification technology has evolved into a viable, functional, clinical treatment modality. It is currently being used to treat many types of behavioral disorders. Operant behavior modification technology is based on two key psychological principles that account for the way a resident behaves. They are: 1) reinforcement, and 2) stimulus control. Reinforcement is an incentive concept. It is used to motivate the resident to do what nursing home personnel feel he or she must do to make progress during the treatment process. Stimulus control accounts for why a particular pattern of behavior will occur in a particular context.

The key concept that ties those two principles together to make it possible to teach the resident is the reinforcement contingency. It combines the reinforcement and stimulus control principle together by a very specific contractual arrangement. Fox, for example, "states that if a trainer instructs a resident, an elderly man, in training in a dressing program, to get completely dressed, including putting on his underpants, pants, shirt, socks and shoes, all in a very specific manner, within a specified time limit, he could have his breakfast -- this would be a reinforcement contingency."

The main treatment vehicle used in the operant system is the contingent reinforcement approach combined with a set of teaching procedures called Programmed instruction. Basically, behavior is a task analyzed into "teachable units," i.e., units that are suitable for the particular population of interest. The units are designed so that the residents appropriate attention to learning the steps that make up the particular skill is maintained as much as possible or at their present level. Attention is controlled through promoting and fading techniques. All of this sequencing of programming is done on a contingent reinforcement basis.

The objective of this book is to encourage the reader to begin to focus on treatment strategies in terms of measurable behavioral deficits when providing care for the elderly rather than on the somewhat nebulous concept of "old age". It follows that those either, 1) fail to exhibit certain basic skills of behaviors or 2) they exhibit to an excessive degree certain behaviors society labels as being maladaptive, obnoxious, immature, stereotyped or disruptive.

Further, it focuses on the use of empirically grounded behavioral privileges that maladaptive behavior is learned, and is not fundamentally different from any maladaptive behavior. In particular, it exists because of the residents learning history, current interaction with his or her environment and/or loss of cognitive skills. The traditional "intra-psychic" process and motives are presumed to be nonexistent and is not needed or useful in behavior programming.

The first part of this book will be aimed towards providing basic behavior training techniques to those healthcare professionals who provide those basic, direct, hands-on services to those residents who have experienced significant skill loss in routine hygiene and personal care activities. The second part will be devoted to procedure designed to eliminate specified behaviors which have been classified as maladaptive inappropriate and/or "problem behaviors."

Finally, the purpose of this book is to provide parents, family members, teachers, and the healthcare providers who work in nursing homes and long term care facilities how to effectively use behavior modification techniques in their treatment strategies. Behavior programming is a field tested reliable and psycho educational approach to treatment of the elderly with Alzheimer's dementia.

In conclusion the material provides basic guiding principles to be followed -- that residents be trained to function as normally as he or she can within the segment of society in which they reside or to which they will return. And in doing so, it is assumed that the staff will use good professional judgment in determining the manner in which they respond to the behavior of the residents and use common sense in developing all behavioral programming.

CHAPTER ONE

BRIDGING ACTIVITIES
A MATTER OF PERSPECTIVE

Bridging is a term the author uses to emphasize the delicate relationship of trust between the elderly in need of skilled nursing home care, their caregiver and nursing home personnel. Bridging is an exercise of discipline on the part of anyone and everyone involved in the admissions process and treatment of the elderly. Bridging is a complex task requiring flexibility, balance, and good judgment in programming. Bridging mandates that both the caregiver and nursing home personnel deliver mature mental health techniques in the decision making process. Bridging demands an extraordinary capacity on the part of the family members and caregivers in the nursing home to flexibly explore and continually examine and re-examine the delicate balance between conflicting needs, goals, objectives, strategies and responsibilities of all parties concerned. Bridging is then a discipline because it is an act of giving up something we feel that is important or a series of losses which are painful. Bridging is that relationship that grows out of the emotional give and take on the part of the resident, caregiver and nursing home community alike.

When one begins to seriously examine activity programs in today's nursing homes, one finds programming to be little if any different from programs in previous generations in the industry. In far too many instances commonly held stereotypes are unconsciously fostered and encouraged. In fact, because we are now talking about an essentially captive group of individuals, the elderly, with health problems and values who have relatively few alternatives, it becomes easy for us to continue prescribing activities which have little therapeutic value.

In far too many instances, the philosophy of most activity programs have been one of keeping the residents busy with the sole objective of having fun.

One would certainly not want to suggest that there is not value in having fun; however, one wonders just how many of us would be content to spend all of our time merely having fun, or pursuing the pleasure principle in life.

By conducting activity programs whose primary purpose is keeping residents occupied and having pleasant experiences, we are implying a great deal to the participants. What we are saying to them, with a program which consists mainly of recreationally oriented group activities requiring little, if any, interaction such as arts and crafts, parties, entertainment, and bingo is that our philosophy is one of play.

The purpose of an activity program in today's Nursing Home Facility is to create as near to a normal environment as possible. An adequate activity program has been described, by most professionals in the discipline, as the involvement of all residents in the facility in some type of program in which they are interested individually, and which meet their physical, competitive, mental, emotional, social and spiritual needs on a daily basis. An activity program in a long-term care facility means the conscious management of daily life through creating, supporting, developing, and restoring the appropriate life-style of the resident in the direction of personal and social autonomy. Activity programming does not mean just recreation, but everything and anything that happens in the life of a resident including all the interaction in which he or she is engaged.

Such definitions begin to suggest something far different from what has become the rather traditional nursing home activity program. They suggest all programming should be therapeutic in nature. They suggest that the basic concern is for the quality of life of the resident and on how he or she spends their days. They suggest that while group recreational activities are a part of the program, they should not be the whole and that they too can be therapeutic addressing social interaction, participation, exercise, improving fine and gross motor and cognitive skills.

The kind of activity program which is presently being emphasized must involve every staff member in the facility. This implies that the activity director is more of a coordinator rather than a director, planning so that the resident's individual needs are met while at the same time insuring a team approach and continuity of care is maintained throughout the process.

The prime concern of any activity program is to help the individual resident to take part in as full, meaningful, and satisfying day of which he or she is capable. This includes the resident who is capable of spending most of his or her day in individual and group activities as well as the resident who is bedfast, confused, demented or those who have over-lapping psychological disorders. The resident should be helped to utilize his or her abilities, regardless of how limited, to achieve meaning, satisfaction, and fun as well as modifying inappropriate behavior and skill loss. This suggests the kind of activity program which has as many different kinds of opportunities as possible with as few limitations as possible.

Having suggested all of this, one could make the assumption that such a philosophy suggests a utopia situation in which activity personnel would have the time, staff, and financial resources necessary to conduct such an ambitious activity program. In a way this is true if one holds steadfast to the old philosophy of play. In reality, most facilities are already doing much of what is being recommended. However, with some creativity and thinking "outside the box", i.e. the utilization of all the staff, accepting the fact that everything and anything a resident does throughout the day can be an activity and can be programmed as such, the concept of a team approach and continuity of care, such a philosophy has the potential to result in an approach in which each resident will find meaning, satisfaction and a sense of well being. It is the only approach that will insure a team concept and continuity of care.

An activity program which accents such a philosophy can be extremely effective in the management of two major losses which the elderly experience during the aging process: (1) skill loss, especially if they are experiencing dementia or Alzheimer's disease, including those extremely important skills of activities of daily living which include toileting, grooming, dressing and dining. And, (2) inappropriate behavior which generally consists of agitation, non-compliance, inappropriate sexual remarks, exposing themselves, masturbation, voroism, grabbing and fondling others, to name but a few. An activity program can do much to address these behaviors which are a challenge to family members and other caregivers alike. Activity programming should, when relating to such problems, focus in a positive way upon assisting the resident to improve by learning, unlearning, or relearning appropriate behavior and/or at least upon maintaining their present level of functioning.

Such a positive approach of focusing upon teaching specific skills can drastically improve one's view of the elderly changing especially those with dementia or Alzheimer's disease, from a negative stance to a positive one. Our frustration and pessimism is minimized once we see a resident learning, unlearning, or relearning skills or appropriate behavior. The requirements for a resident's learning to occur are: (1) an affective teaching technique and (2) targeting what we should teach. There is no point spending time teaching skills which an individual can do just as well without.

The contents of this book focus on bridging activities of daily living. It contains examples of lesson plans which address most of the daily skills of the elderly who reside in our various health care facilities. These teaching procedures when included in activity programming can result in a wide range of change in the nature of an activity program when implemented in a nursing home or other health care facilities.

The basic procedures for teaching such skills with these lesson plans evolve from two basic principles. They are: (1) reinforcement: praise with physical, verbal and gestural responses when the resident performs a task in a positive manner, and (2) teach all tasks in small, simple steps.

In summary, then, we must begin any and all activities for a reason. We must begin thinking how an activity will help a resident - physically, mentally, emotionally, and spiritually. We must begin thinking about activities based upon the needs and interests of each individual resident. We must pursue a program of activities which is basically concerned with promoting the quality of life of each individual resident. We must mandate that all personnel involved in a resident's habilitation and care, regardless of their discipline and training, be an active participant in the process. And finally, we must bridge past activity programs with future programming. We can do so if we are flexible, use good judgment and strive to achieve a balance between the past, present and future. We may not need to change any activity in which our residents are presently participating. We do need, however, to change our philosophy from one of strictly play or recreation to one which is therapeutic with an understanding that any activity can be adjusted to address a therapeutic need.

CHAPTER TWO

A BEHAVIORAL APPROACH TO TRAINING

The material contained in this book focuses on and adheres to the principles and philosophy of the behavioral model treatment techniques, and strategies of behavior modification. Behaviorists and health care providers alike have found behavior modification to be an effective tool in the treatment of the elderly residing in Nursing Homes and Long Term Care Facilities. In fact it is often the preferred method of treatment by many healthcare professionals providing services for the elderly with dementia and Alzheimer's disease in this population.

Behavior modification is a teaching procedure; it does not attempt to explain old age, and associated illnesses such as dementia and Alzheimer's disease. The aim of behavior modification is a positive one of producing improvement, rather than a passive one of observing, interrupting, and explaining. A case of dementia or Alzheimer's disease is not considered "hopeless". The frail elderly who we serve are often sick, confused, and demented with varying degrees of skill loss are capable of learning, unlearning, and relearning. Behavior modification attempts to teach those individuals specific skills. They were lost skills which helped them to function effectively in their environment, and enjoy a broader scope of personal experiences. Behavior modification puts them in a position to continue learning additional valuable skills.

The focus of behavior modification is always upon improvement. No limit is ever placed on what an individual can learn, other than the limits of his or her own rate of progress. Some individuals may progress quickly; others move more slowly, however, all are viewed as being capable of learning. This positive approach of focusing upon teaching specific skills can drastically alter one's view of working with the elderly. This is true when one is working with those "unstable" psychiatric residents, especially those who have suffered from mental illness most of their lives and who may or may not have an overlapping dementia such as Alzheimer's disease. These residents may be frightened with poor impulse control coupled with depression. However, frustration and pessimism is minimized once caregivers see the residents ability to learn, relearn, and unlearn certain skills and/or behaviors - the requirements for this learning to occur is as follows: (1) An effective teaching procedure, which is provided by behavior modification techniques and (2) deciding what should be taught, should be guided by considerations of practicality and relevance.

In order to ensure practicality, teaching goals must always be limited to what seems meaningful at the point and time the assessment is done at which time his or her needs are established and prioritized. Although long-term goals might be quite ambitious, immediate goals must be more modest. For example, a hyperactive resident may pace actively about his/her living area all day and night. From their personal history, it may appear that they can learn to read, but obviously, to include them in a reading class in such a hyperactive state would be completely impractical. Therefore, an initial practical goal should be to teach the resident to sit in a chair for an assigned number of minutes.

Decisions about the practicality of a particular teaching goal should always be based upon such natural hierarchies. There are certain behavioral prerequisites which have to be taught first. For example, to teach a resident to name colors, he or she must first be taught to look at the colors. Also, to teach a resident to assemble a puzzle, he or she must first be taught to work at a simple task for more than a few seconds. Therefore, one must always start with the basics and gradually build up to a more difficult and elaborate task. By beginning with the things that are the simplest and/or the easiest or most essential to accomplish, other higher-level tasks will become possible.

When considering relevance one must view behavior as being those that will be useful or rewarding to the resident in his or her living environment.

In general, the most relevant behaviors are those which concern daily living skills such as toileting, grooming, dressing, and dining. So long as the resident remains in training and/or teaching environment, skills which will facilitate further learning are relevant. For those residents needing long term skilled care in a Nursing Home providing special care for dementia or Alzheimer's disease it is important to develop behaviors which allow the resident to learn or at least, maintain those skills which are needed and beneficial.

The particular behavior which is targeted to be taught on the basis of these considerations, must be specifically defined clearly and precisely. If what is to be achieved is not specified, little if anything can be achieved. Objectives are an essential first step for any successful treatment plan.

The principles, philosophy and methods of behavior modification must begin by training residents. The principles and training techniques of behavior modification at the facility are based on two facts. (1) All behavior is caused. It is important that all caregiver personnel realize that there are causes for any and all behavior. (2) Behavior is not a permanent or a characteristic of an individual. It can be changed, if the causes can be defined and targeted. This means there is hope for improvement if: (1) the staff is properly trained and has the patience to search for and try to alter the causes of the behavior and (2) the primary cause of current behavior is its past consequences. This directs attention to a specifically defined and major cause of behavior which can be targeted and changed in order to accomplish therapeutic gains.

The success of behavior modification relies upon careful attention to and arrangement of the consequences for behavior occurs mainly because of the effects which it produces. Learning, or any change in behavior, is most easily produced by careful arrangement of the consequences of behavior. It is on this simple fact that behavior modification is established.

Recognition that the most immediate cause of behavior is some character-istic of the environment and/or situation rather than of some characteristic inside the individual opens up the hope of substantial behavioral improvement for the resident. The situation can be so arranged so that it becomes a teaching tool. The relation between a behavior and its consequences is called a contingency, a specification of what leads to what. Therefore, it is mainly through the arrangement of proper contingencies that behavioral changes are accomplished.

The simplest way of defining just what is involved in the behavioral modification process is that one should reward desirable behavior and refrain from rewarding undesirable behavior. Behavior which is rewarded and/or reinforced tends to be repeated, while behavior which is not rewarded tends not to be repeated. This is the heart and soul of teaching behavior modification in that it guarantees that desirable behavior has reinforcing effects, and that undesirable behavior does not.

There are two types of goals which are used by practitioners in implementing behavior modification techniques. The first goal is teaching and/or training the resident some new and appropriate behaviors. The second goal is to eliminate types of undesirable and/or inappropriate behavior which a resident is exhibiting. For example, one goal may be to teach or train a resident how to dress him or herself without staff assistance, while on the other hand he or she may be taught to eliminate the behavior of hitting others. In both instances, teaching and eliminating behavior with such procedures depend upon the scheduling of appropriate consequences to behavior.

When behavior modification programming is first introduced into a facility, the rules of the caregiver change. Behavior modification is not simply providing a new or better way for the staff to do their job. The staff's role changes from a caregiver to one of a trainer or teacher. Often the main job of the staff in a nursing home or long term care facility has been providing special levels of care for the resident with paternalistic ways of doing things and/or tasks for them and to them. Under such circumstances the residents learn little, if any, desirable skills or behavior much less being taught how to maintain useful skills. In fact, the behavioral deterioration and skill loss often is a result of chronic institutionalization in long term care facilities. Much of the worst behavior seen in residents develops following their admission to a facility. Little thought is given to outplacement into a less restrictive setting in the community. Therefore, a thorough behavior modification program can result in a wide-ranging change in the nature and philosophy of long term care facilities.

In teaching behavior modification, skill training programming employ shaping procedures where each behavior or skill is broken down into a simple chain of sub-behaviors, behavior components, stages, or steps.

Each behavioral component in a chain will constitute a stage for training and data recording purposes. The programs are written with the stages broken down as minutely as possible into small, simple steps so that the least difficult task may be selected for training. The program outline should be followed closely, stage by stage and step by step, especially with those residents who are more resistant to the training process. In some cases, however, a resident may demonstrate that he or she can complete more of the sequences than the stage or step being taught. If this occurs, the trainer can combine two or more steps for training purposes but for data reporting purposes, each step should be reported on separately.

When the resident has met the criterion for a step, he or she will begin training on the next new step, but will be required to repeat the previously learned sequences of steps learned as well as the new step in order to pass that stage. The process involved is called backward chaining. This is where the behavioral sequence, for training purposes, begins with the last step in the chain and progresses toward completion of the entire sequence of training in reverse order requiring the resident to complete the previously learned step and chain the sequence into a forward or natural order of occurrence.

SHAPING AND REINFORCEMENT:

The shaping procedures to be employed will involve reinforcing successful backward approximations to the sequence within a stage. This will be accomplished by the trainer withdrawing all physical assistance toward the end of the behavioral chain. The resident can then complete the task him or herself, thus performing a successive approximation to the terminal behavior. Reinforcement (reward) will be given only for successful completion of a part of the behavioral chain, with the trainer requiring the resident to complete more and more of the behavior of the chain on his or her own as training progresses before reinforcement and or reward is given. More specifically, a trial consists of the following sequences.

1. A command from the trainer.
2. A brief pause by the trainer to allow resident time to respond.
3. Trainer gives resident graduated guidance and/or modeling.
4. Trainer gives reinforcement for successful approximations the trainer will Set up the training situation as outlines for each stage and/or step of a Program and then gives the appropriate command in a kind, firm, clear and empathetic voice. If the resident does not begin responding upon Command, the trainer should immediately physically assist the resident to complete the behavior or the trainer should immediately model the desired behavior for the resident to initiate and then physically assist to completion if the resident does not respond. Each time, assistance is withdrawn just prior to the completion of the behavior.

Upon successful completion of the stage or step, reinforcement is given. A tangible or edible reinforcer will be something that the resident has demonstrated that he or she prefers or likes to do or to eat i.e., potato chips, ice cream, candy, T.V., etc. Social reinforcement should always be given. i.e., a hug, pat on the back or good boy or good girl comments, etc. As training progresses, edible reinforcers should be gradually faded out by softening the tone of voice when giving resident a command. In any case, edibles should be given in very small quantities to avoid satiation.

Training data should be reported on following each individual trial and recorded. In order to receive a plus on the data sheet, the resident must correctly perform the entire behavior component of a stage without assistance. If the resident attempts to make the response but has to be assisted, then, he or she receives a minus on the data sheet. If she or he makes no effort at all and/or resists shaping so that the response fails to occur, then, he or she receives a zero on the data sheet. An equally acceptable and more realistic alternative is to a periodic weekly test and report on the highest stage or step passed. This test may be accomplished by beginning with the terminal step in the program and, working in a backward order, testing each step until one is reached which the resident successfully completes. In order to move from one step to another, however, the trainer must at least record a plus for each step passed on the data sheet. The criteria for passing a step should be nineteen correct responses out of the previous twenty attempted prior to the time of evaluation. The training sessions should last no longer than fifteen minutes per individual resident, or until the resident demonstrates his or her ability to successfully pass each step of the program. In this event, sessions should be discontinued until a later time or until a rest period has elapsed.

When the resident has successfully completed the program by responding correctly to all the steps including the terminal one which ends the training, the trainer will begin fading the prompts and continue fading reinforcement and place the resident on a maintenance schedule. During the maintenance period the resident should now be required to perform the newly learned behavior on his or her own at an appropriately scheduled time and place. The trainer will continue the monitoring and/or shaping process in a natural setting until the resident no longer has to be commanded to perform the behavior and when reinforcements, other than social ones, are no longer needed. Periodically, however, the resident should receive social reinforcement each day for performing or for having performed the behavior. For example, after the resident has learned to put on his or her socks or hose the trainer sees that he or she continues the behavior learned by putting his or her socks or hose on by him or herself each morning.

GRADUATED GUIDANCE:

Graduated guidance is used in behavior modification to teach residents skills who have lost cognitive abilities or who has difficulty understanding the instructor. This technique involves simply manually guiding the resident through the proper motions with the amount of hand pressure adjusted from moment to moment dependent upon the performance of the resident at the time in learning a task. The following procedures should be adhered to when implementing graduated guidance when training a resident.

1. Use no more than minimal demands needed to make the resident begin performing the desired behavior. The trainer should begin by using the least amount of pressure possible and build up the pressure until the resident begins to move.

2. Once the behavior is in progress, the trainer should begin immediately to gradually decrease the guidance. The trainer continues to decrease guidance as long as the resident continues to perform the desired behavior.

3. If the resident stops performing the task during a trial, the trainer immediately increases guidance gradually to a point where he or she is performing the task again.

4. If the resident resists guidance by pushing against the trainer in the direction away from the proper motions required by the behavior apply just enough guidance to counter-act the resident's resistance. The goal is to stop the resident from resisting, although he or she may still be exhibiting non-compliance.

5. As the resident decreases the degree of opposing the guidance, the trainer instantly decreases his or her commands so that the resident's resistance is counterbalanced again.

6. When the resistance ceases, the trainer immediately, but gradually, uses just enough guidance to start the behavior again.

7. Once the trainer begins a trial, he or she will continue to use graduated guidance until the response has been completed; the trainer should not give up or interrupt before the final step.

There are two procedures which constitute the next lower level of guidance to be used once guidance has been faded to a mere touch: (1) shadowing and (2) spatial fading. In shadowing, the trainer's hand follows the residents hand or whatever body parts that is being involved in the behavior, of a distance of a fraction of an inch without touching the resident. Spatial fading, which is an alternative method that may be used to fade out touch contact, involves moving the touch contact away from the focal point of the behavior is to pick up an object with the hand (focal point), the trainer should move contact back to the wrist, the forearm, the elbow, the upper arm, and then to the shoulder and back within each trial.

MODELLING:

Modelling is also used in teaching residents. This procedure is used with residents who have demonstrated that they can imitate a model. This means that the trainer demonstrates each step by actually doing it him or herself. The trainer will give the command and immediately performs the desired sequence of behavior him or herself. If the resident fails to imitate the trainer then he or she must be physically assisted to do so by the trainer using graduated guidance to perform the desired behavior. However, if the resident is able to imitate the trainer's behavior, the trainer will immediately reinforce the resident and proceed to the next step in the training procedure. If at any point during the procedure the resident fails to attempt to imitate, the trainer will physically assist the resident in making the response and socially reinforce him or her.

PROMPTS AND COMMANDS:

Prompts and commands are vital in implementing behavior modification and teaching behavior skills. A prompt is either a verbal or gestural cue that tells the resident that the trainer wants him or her to do something. Verbal prompts consist of instructions of commands while gestural prompts usually consist of pointing, looking toward a particular spot or direction, or touching the resident, etc. During the initial part of training, prompts should be given quite often on a regular basis. During the final stages of training, a great deal of care must be taken to use the least amount of prompting necessary at every stage or step. This process is much more rapid with residents who have maintained their cognitive skills as prompting is usually necessary only in the very beginning. Residents who have declining cognitive skills, however, need prompting for longer periods of time, especially when they are taught a complex chain of behaviors.

A major problem with prompting is that the resident may become dependent on the trainer and the prompts instead of performing the behavior on his or her own. It becomes necessary to fade prompts as quickly as possible so that the residents will perform on his or her own in the absence of the trainer.

Prompts vary in the degree of information available to the resident. The more active and conspicuous or the more information given, the less reason the resident has to rely on his or her memory and motivation. Fading dependency should be accomplished by fading prompts, by giving a less active prompt than was given on the proceeding trial. For example, when a resident is prompted to go to the toilet, the trainer may touch him or her on the shoulder, point to the toilet, and give verbal instructions. On the next trial he or she may point only to the toilet and give verbal instructions. The next time, the trainer may reduce part of the verbal instruction until the process progresses to a point where no prompt will be given and the resident will have to decide to self-initiate.

There are two methods of fading prompts: (1) reduce the number of words in a verbal instruction or command, or (2) by gradually softening the tone in which the command is given. Verbal prompts should be faded first and the gestural prompts last since verbal prompts are difficult to fade out gradually. Table 1 is an example of toilet approach prompting with some general guidelines to use in prompting (upper portion) as well as the order in which prompts should be faded (lower portion).The prompts are arranged in order with the most active or conspicuous at the top and decreasing to the least active at the bottom. One should note that reduction of verbal prompts begins as soon as touch contact, graduated guidance, has been eliminated.

TABLE I

PROMPTS USED IN TOILETING

(EXAMPLE)

General Guidelines:

1. Determine the minimal prompt to which the resident responds. This may be a touch, pointing to the toilet, or instruction.
2. Use a less active prompt the next time the resident is prompted to use the toilet.
3. Wait a few seconds after the prompt before giving graduated guidance.
4. The sequence of toileting prompts are listed below from the most active to the least active. The resident will usually begin independently toileting himself before the least active prompt is given.

Sequence of steps:

Prompt	Example
1. Verbal instruction	"Jane, go to the toilet".
Gesture	Point to toilet
Touch	Lightly tug at resident's blouse
	Guide her from her chair to toilet
2. Verbal instructions	"Jane, go to the toilet".
Gesture	Point to toilet
No touch	
3. Reduced verbal instruction	"Jane, toilet".
Gesture	Point to toilet.
No touch	
4. Reduced verbal instruction	"toilet".
Gesture	Point to toilet.
No touch	
5. No verbal instruction	Point to toilet with arm fully extended.
Gesture	Motion toward toilet with head.
No touch	
6. No verbal instruction	Point to toilet with arm
Reduced gesture	Partially extended with full motion.
No touch	
7. No verbal instruction	Point to toilet with full head motion.
Reduced gesture	
No arm motion	
No touch	

8. No verbal introduction	Motion towards toilet with head only.
Reduced gesture	
No touch	

9. No verbal instruction	Move eyes towards toilet only.
Reduced gesture	
No head motion	
No touch	

Once the phase has been reached where slight arm, head, or eye movements are effective, the fading process begins to occur naturally as the trainer's head and arms normally move about in his or her interaction with the resident. The gestural prompt will simply blend into this movement background so that the resident will be less able to depend on the cue value of the trainer's movements and will, instead, begin relying on his or her memory and motivation. Since residents with restricted cognitive skills have difficulty remembering it will probably be necessary to begin training each day with the last prompt that was used successfully on the previous day. The trainer may have to even move back a step in the program to give an even more obvious prompt. One should remember, however, to start with the prompt to which the resident successfully responded on the previous day and/or training session.

REINFORCEMENT:

When implementing any behavior modification program positive reinforcement is vital. Therefore, something of an edible nature is always used as reinforcement as well as anything the resident likes, will approach, and will perform some response to get. Therefore, a good reinforcement plan must be individualized. It may take more time to find out what a resident likes verses what is convenient, but it saves time in the long run. There are a number of ways to define what a resident likes:

1. Take him or her to the dining room and observe what he or she chooses to eat.

2. Ask a family member, friend, relative or significant other who knows or is near him or her most of the time.

3. Observe him or her during dining to see which food and liquids he or she chooses first.

4. Use the trial and error and or baseline by using reinforcement sampling. Offer a large variety of food and drink samples and wait for a positive or negative response during imitation or on command. Observe the resident's approach to the various samples and date his or her enthusiasm or vigor in responding to each reinforcer during the trials.

Some tips to consider in using positive reinforcement are:

1. Find at least two most highly preferred food or drinks. Use the second highest preferred choice when it appears that the resident is satiated on the first.

2. Good reinforcers do not take long to consume. Liquids, soft foods, chocolate candy, potato chips and French fries are good when given in small amounts. They should always be fresh and consult medical staff before implementing.

3. Good reinforcers should be broken down into small servings and or bites for:
   A. Quick consumption
   B. To avoid satiation
   C. To minimize nutritional defects over a period of time.

4. Individualize training time to avoid least interference with meal's effects.

5. Consider possible medical or dental consequences with prolonged use of any reinforcer.

FADING REINFORCEMENT:

In the initial stages of any training program, continuous reinforcement is given. This means that the trainer reinforces every successful attempt or successive approximation. As training progresses, however, and the resident begins to come under control of the command or stimulus, reinforcement should be faded, gradually reduced, until a point is reached at which the trainer will no longer give reinforcement, i.e., the behavior will be completely under control of the command, stimulus or until this is also faded.

The trainer, in consultation with professional and medical personnel, will have to use his or her own judgment as to just how rapidly and how much to fade reinforcement. As an example, however, the trainer might begin by reinforcing every trial and, then when the behavior comes under stimulus control, start fading by reinforcing on every trial, every fifth trial, etc., and finally, for perhaps on average of ten trials. The ultimate goal to work toward is zero reinforcement given by the trainer.

The procedure simply involves requiring the resident to do more and more each time for reinforcement. This can involve having the resident perform it correctly a greater number of times before reinforcers are given, or it may involve having the resident perform more of the task itself, i.e., more parts of a behavioral chain. In a skill training program, the first stage or step may be reinforced on continuous reinforcement program. For example, the second stage or step may also begin on a continuous reinforcement schedule. Then, at some point during the second stage of learning the resident should not be given reinforcement unless he or she performs both stages or steps of one and two to completion, while the trainer drops reinforcement for just performing stage two. If it becomes apparent that the trainer has required too much of the resident before reinforcement is given, then the trainer should drop back to the point where the behavior was previously under control with a certain amount of reinforcement being given. Then the trainer should gradually continue the fading process.

If this training methodology seems similar to those used in teaching children - it is. When training children during their formative years we do so by teaching a task over and over. Children learn by repetitive performances and rewarded for positive results, they are never rewarded for negative performance. The difference in training a child versus the elderly is that a child's cognitive skills are growing and developing while cognitive skills are declining among the elderly, making it more difficult to train the elderly resident. The best we can expect, as trainers, is to help the elderly maintain their present level of skills they presently possess and to hopefully slow further skill loss and reduce maladaptive behavior.

CHAPTER THREE

TRAINING AND ABUSE

There are two elements of concern which are worrisome to caregivers charged with meeting the physical, mental, emotional and spiritual needs of the elderly residing in a nursing home facility. They are: Loss of daily living activities in the vital areas of toileting, grooming, dressing and dining and exhibiting inappropriate and/or maladaptive behavior. Therefore, based on the assumption that these individuals can continue to learn, unlearn and relearn lost skills it is imperative that training programs be implemented, to at least, assist the elderly resident to maintain their present level of skills. It is important that these residents receive the <u>right help,</u> at the <u>right time</u> from the <u>right person</u> at the <u>right facility</u>. It is also imperative that caregivers involved in the formal training process of these residents examine their own feelings, beliefs and more specifically their attitudes about how they relate to abuse, its nature and its causes. It is necessary for caregivers to examine their philosophy of caring for the elderly because abuse on any level almost always has a powerful impact on the ability of the caregiver to provide adequate, appropriate meaningful training to those residents with skill loss and maladaptive behavior.

When we consider training the elderly in the areas of activities of daily living in geriatric settings we must remember that abuse can occur during the training process. It can be problematic, for a number of reasons, both on the part of the resident, the caregiver, or both. For example, abuse can occur if the resident does not feel good, is demented, restless, or hyperactive, making it difficult for him or her to understand and follow directions. Therefore, caregivers who function as trainers must always remember that the elderly population are often frail, sick, confused, and lonely and feel helpless, all which are present barriers to any type of training. Also, there are times when the resident exhibits episodes of inappropriate behavior which makes it impossible to train him or her due to their aggressiveness, anger or disruptive behavior. Then too, there are times when the caregiver who does the training reports comes to work tired, upset, angry, and/or depressed along with a litany of other family, personal or dysfunctional events in their lives which in an institutional environment is not conducive to training.

However, such events should not make training a behavioral nightmare. Training should be rescheduled at a later time when both the resident and trainer are able to participate in the training procedures as scheduled. It is better to postpone a training exercise than risk the possibility of abuse. It is essential that all training be done in a healthy training environment conducive to the needs of the resident. Consideration must always be given to the welfare of the resident realizing that abuse is an ongoing challenge that deserves critical attention, continued surveillance and creative solutions. Although training is vital it should not be done at the expense of the resident.

Demanding too much from a resident can create problems for those with cognitive difficulties especially those with dementia and Alzheimer's disease. Many caregivers feel they need to develop activity programs which exercise a resident's brain -- training every hour of everyday pushing them to achieve. Such demands are unnerving for a family member or a caregiver in an institution involved in training exercises to observe a resident who is struggling, making mistakes and is unable to correct them. However, targeting and addressing such needs in training programs are necessary. Training is essential to help the resident learn, unlearn and relearn skills and behavior. Here are some pointers:

First - think about how you feel when someone tells you that you have made a mistake before God and Country. Being corrected makes anyone feel intimidated. The resident with memory loss is constantly being confronted with their mistakes, which makes them feel at a loss and extremely uncomfortable. What we need to do as a caregiver during a training session is make the resident comfortable with the knowledge and/or skill level they have - as long as they are in a safe and comfortable environment.

Second - Don't overtax their brain. It is not a muscle and should not be exercised as such. A resident with memory loss is not lazy. He or she has a disability that is, in many ways, like an amputation. As a caregiver, we have to assume the resident is working as hard as they can at any given moment with the abilities that he or she has left at a particular time. Residents with memory loss have good and bad days. As a caregiver, we have to accept the resident's changing cognitive abilities each day, each hour and each minute as the best the resident can do right now, at this moment, and at his or her point and time.

Third - We must, as a caregiver, avoid quizzing or asking a resident a specific or pointed question such as "Do you remember me"? "What is your name?", "Do you remember what we did yesterday?". For a resident, life becomes like a constant test when they have memory loss and we as caregivers don't want them to feel as if they have that test over and over.

Fourth - If the resident becomes upset we should try to distract them, redirecting them to another and quite area rather than correcting or confronting them. If this effort doesn't work we should, after we make sure the resident is safe, walk away and let them calm down.

Fifth - We should not in our role as a caregiver announce things or activities in advance. Residents with memory loss have problems figuring out time sequences. They become upset and fearful about schedules -- especially a physicians visit or appointment. Any activity should be announced at the last possible moment.

Sixth - Let the resident forget. If we as a caregiver lose our tempers if he or she refuses a bath, or has an inappropriate behavioral outburst, we should ignore or leave the resident alone and approach him or her again later. By that time the resident will have forgotten what was upsetting them.

Seventh - If the resident has forgotten how to perform an activity we as a caregiver should assist them with it. The caregiver should never try to "talk the resident through the activity", or have them struggle "thinking about how to do it". Thinking about it only worsens the problem. Redirection should be done instead. Redirection is simply changing the subject. Examples include: Moving on to another task; giving the resident a glass of juice or liquid of choice, making a phone call to a friend, looking at a family or familiar picture in an album, or reading a letter aloud. We as a caregiver should let the resident's memory loss work for us. If a letter, joke, or other method is helpful once, we should not be afraid to use it over and over.

And finally, if we as caregivers adhere to these points when interacting with a resident in our charge using careful observation, patience, and consistency, we should be able to avoid the many risk factors in training which might be interpreted as abuse.

CHAPTER FOUR

DRESSING PROGRAM

This chapter addresses the area of human behavior in which the elderly or those suffering from Alzheimer's Disease experience varying degrees of skill loss in dressing. The purpose of the development of these examples of Training Programs in dressing is to provide parents, teachers, family members and more specifically the Healthcare provider in Nursing Home Facilities how to use behavior modification techniques to observe, measure, change and manage behavior in a humane fashion based on the principles of operant conditioning. The examples stated in this chapter are approved methods of modifying behavior and are practical, detailed and easy to implement. The objective of this program is to teach or train the resident to learn, unlearn, relearn, and/or to at least maintain existing skills at their present level in dressing.

TABLE OF CONTENTS

DRESSING SKILLS ASSESSMENT

Resident_____ No. _____ Date _____

Evaluator _____Living Area _____

Rating:

1. Never been observed to perform the skill by him or herself even though he or she has had the opportunity.

2. Does it sometimes by him or herself, but not adequately (slowly, because he or she <u>does not know</u> - this means that you have never seen him or her do it correctly at least once, but he or she tries).

3. Performs skill adequately with verbal prompts (if someone tells him or her to do it or how to do it).

4. Does it sometimes by him or herself but not adequately (sloppy, but he or she does know how - this means that you have seen him or her do it correctly at least once).

5. Performs skill adequately and consistently (most of the time) without verbal, gestural or physical prompting.

6. No opportunity to perform skill.

7. P.D. Does not perform - physically disabled.

SKILL	RATING 1-8
1. Puts on bra	_____
2. Takes off bra	_____
3. Puts on socks	_____
4. Takes off socks	_____
5. Puts on hose	_____
6. Takes off hose	_____
7. Puts on panty hose	_____
8. Takes off panty hose	_____
9. Puts on t-shirt	_____
10. Takes off t-shirt	_____
11. Puts on pants	_____
12. Takes off pants	_____
13. Puts on underpants	_____
14. Takes off underpants	_____

D-2 SKILL   RATING 1-7

15. Puts on dress   _____

16. Takes off dress   _____

17. Puts on skirt   _____

18. Takes off skirt   _____

19. Puts on slip   _____

20. Takes off slip   _____

21. Puts on coat   _____

22. Takes off coat   _____

23. Puts on button-down shirt/blouse _____

24. Takes off button-down shirt/blouse _____

25. Puts on hat/cap   _____

26. Takes off hat/cap   _____

27. Puts on shoe   _____

28. Takes off shoe   _____

29. Puts on boot   _____

30. Takes off boot   _____

31. Puts on gloves   _____

32. Takes off gloves   _____

33. Zipping   _____

34. Unzipping   _____

35. Buttoning   _____

36. Unbuttoning   _____

37. Snapping   _____

38. Unsnapping   _____

39. Tying   _____

40. Untying   _____

41. Puts on belt   _____

42. Takes off belt   _____

43. Puts on tie   _____

44. Takes off tie   _____

45. Hooks bra   _____

46. Unhooks bra   _____

47. Recognizes own clothing   _____

48. Selects correct clothes for specific event   _____

49. Selects correct clothes for social events   _____

D-3 SKILL   RATING 1-7

50. Recognizes dirty clothing   _____

51. Can change clothes when dirty   _____

52. Can change clothes when torn   _____

53. Wears neatly pressed clothing   _____

54. Matches color combinations   _____

55. Differentiates between work/dress clothes _____

56. Differentiates between work/dress shoes   _____

57. Hangs pants on hanger   _____

58. Hangs dress on hanger   _____

59. Places shoes in closet, beneath bed   _____

60. Puts clothing in proper storage place   _____

61. Folds towels/ sheets   _____

62. Make complete change of clothing from
one activity to another.   _____

63. Opens umbrella   _____

64. Closes umbrella   _____

65. Folds shirts/blouse for storage   _____

66. Folds pants for storage   _____

67. Folds towels/sheets   _____

68. Puts folded clothes away properly   _____

69. Places dirty clothes in correct place   _____

70. Washes clothing by hand   _____

71. Wash clothing by machine   _____

72. Sorts clothing for washing   _____

73. Irons clothes   _____

Dressing Training Order D-4
DRESS

MALE	FEMALE or	FEMALE
1. T-shirt	1. Bra	1. Bra
2. Underpants	2. Panties	2. Blouse
3. Shirt	3. Slip	3. Panties
4. Pants	4. Dress	4. Pants/skirt
5. Sock	5. Sock/hose	5. Sock
6. Shoe	6. Shoe	6. Shoe

UNDRESS

MALE	FEMALE or	FEMALE
1. Shoe	1. Shoe	1. Shoe
2. Sock	2. Sock/hose	2. Sock/hose
3. Pants	3. Dress	3. Pants/skirt
4. Shirt	4. Slip	4. Blouse
5. Underpants	5. Panties	5. Panties
6. T-shirt	6. Bra	6. Bra

CLOTHES TRAINING

Beginning with the second skill taught in the above sequences, requires the resident to perform all the dressing skills he or she has learned. The command will be "JOHN, TAKE OFF YOUR CLOTHES", or "JOHN, PUT ON YOUR CLOTHES". Each time John learns a new skill, add it to the requirement to take off his clothes, or to put on his clothes. For example, in the undressing sequence, suppose you have taught John to take off his shoes and socks. After John learns to take off his shoes, he must then take off his socks. After John learns to take off his pants, he must then take off his shoes, socks, and pants, in that order, and so on for the other skills, in response to the command to take off his clothes. In the dressing sequence, add a step in which John tucks his shirt into his pants.

Keep a separate data sheet for CLOTHES-UNDRESSING AND DRESSING. Use the numbers of the sequences above to enter the data. For example, in the undressing sequence, enter step 1 if John has learned to take off his shoes. Enter step 2 if he is working on taking off his shoes and socks in response to the command to take off his clothes. Enter step 3 in response to the command to take off his clothes. Enter step 4 if he is working on taking off his shoes, socks, and pants, and so on. In doing the actual training it is necessary to point to his shoes and then to his socks and so on to get John to take both articles off. The trainer might also couple the commands for the separate skills with the new command in the beginning, but then begin fading out the old command in favor of clothes.

MODEL LESSON 001
TASK: PUTTING ON BRA.

GOAL: Improve dressing skills.

OBJECTIVE: To teach Jane to put on her bra without assistance.

MATERIALS: Bra of Jane's normal size.

SETTING: Jane sits or stands, the trainer stands near her.

PRE/TEST-POST/TEST: Begin with bra placed front down on Jane's lap.

The trainer touches bra and says, "Jane, put on your bra".

Attention: Do not reinforce a correct response and do not correct an incorrect response - give no assistance.

TEACHING PROCEDURE

Step 1: Use proper size bra for Jane. Begin with bra off Jane. The trainer puts the bra on Jane and hooks it in the back so that Jane's left arm is through the left strap with the strap resting on Jane's mid-arm just above the elbow; the cups should be positioned so that it will fall into place when the strap is pulled up. Trainer touches the bra and says, "JANE, PUT ON YOUR BRA", and immediately assists Jane to grasp the left strap with her right thumb and forefinger and to pull up onto her shoulder. The cup should fall into place; if not, Jane can be assisted to position bra properly. Repeat similar action, giving the same command, with the right strap.

STEP 2: Begin with bra off Jane. The trainer puts bra partially on Jane by hooking it in the back so that the left strap is hanging off Jane's wrists. The right strap is off Jane, hanging loose. The trainer touches Jane's bra and says, "JANE, PUT ON YOUR BRA," and immediately assists Jane to grasp the left strap with her right thumb and forefinger and pull it to the elbow. Jane should complete action learned in step 1. Repeat similar action with right strap so that bra falls into place.

STEP 3: Begin with bra off Jane. The trainer puts bra partially on Jane and hooks bra in the back, so that the straps are hanging off toward her waist. The trainer touches bra strap and says, "JANE, PUT ON YOUR BRA", and immediately assists Jane to grasp the left strap with her right thumb and forefinger and put her wrist through the strap. Perform similar action with right hand. Jane should complete action to position bra properly.

STEP 4: Begin with bra off Jane. The trainer puts bra on Jane so that the cups are on Jane's lower back with straps hanging towards waist, bra is hooked. The trainer touches bra and says, "JANE, PUT ON YOUR BRA", and immediately assists Jane to pull around to the position described in step 3. Jane should complete the action to position bra properly.

STEP 5: Begin with bra off Jane. The trainer puts hook end of bra in Jane's appropriate hand and holds it on Jane's stomach. The trainer touches bra and says, "JANE, PUT ON YOUR BRA," and assists Jane to take the appropriate hand and reach around to her back (clasp end of bra) and grasps the hook end of bra, to pull it around to the front in the proper position, and fasten it. Jane should complete action to position bra properly.

STEP 6: Begin with bra face down near Jane but off Jane, the trainer points to bra and says, "JANE, PUT ON YOUR BRA", and assists Jane to pick up the hook end of bra, to hold it on her stomach, and to reach around behind to grasp the clasp end with the appropriate hand and pull it around to meet the hook end of bra on her stomach. Jane should hook the bra, pull it around properly to the front and complete action to position bra properly.

STEP 7: Terminal behavior, begin with bra face down near Jane. The trainer points toward bra and says, "JANE, PUT ON YOUR BRA". Give minimal reinforcement and assistance as required, gradually fading assistance.

MODEL LESSON 002
TASK: TAKING OFF BRA.

GOAL: Improve dressing skills.

OBJECTIVE: To teach Jane how to take off her bra without assistance.

MATERIALS: A bra sized to fit Jane.

SETTING: Jane and trainer sitting or standing, facing each other.

PRE-TEST/POST-TEST: The trainer puts Jane's bra completely on Jane and says, "JANE, TAKE OFF YOUR BRA." Give no assistance. Do not correct an incorrect response and do not reinforce a correct response.

TEACHING PROCEDURE

STEP 1: Use normal size bra throughout. Begin with hooked bra around Jane's waist with cups on back, straps loose. The trainer says, "JANE, TAKE OFF YOUR BRA." Give no assistance. Do not correct an incorrect response and do not reinforce a correct response.

STEP 2: Use normal size bra throughout. Begin with hooked bra around Jane's waist with cups on back, straps loose. The trainer says, "JANE, TAKE OFF YOUR BRA". And immediately assists Jane to unhook the bra and put it down.

STEP 3: Begin with hooked bra around Jane's waist with cups in front, straps are loose. The trainer says, "JANE, TAKE OFF YOUR BRA," and immediately assists Jane to pull bra around so that cups are on back.

STEP 4: Begin with hooked bra around Jane with straps on wrist. The trainer says, "JANE, TAKE OFF YOUR BRA", and immediately assists Jane to pull bra off the wrists, one at one time.

STEP 5: Repeat step 4 with straps at mid-arm.

STEP 6: Repeat step 4 with straps on shoulders.

STEP 7: Terminal behavior. Give minimal reinforcement and assistance as required, gradually fading assistance.

MODEL LESSON 003
TASK: PUTTING ON SOCK.

GOAL: Improve dressing skills.

OBJECTIVE: To teach the resident to put on his or her sock upon request.

MATERIALS: A nylon stretch sock two sizes too large for the resident; a nylon stretch sock a resident's normal size.

SETTING: Resident and the trainer sitting on the floor, resident with shoes and socks off.

PRE-TEST/POST-TEST: Use normal size sock. Place sock beside the resident's right foot. The trainer touches the sock and says, "JOHN, PUT ON YOUR SOCK". Do not reinforce a correct response and do not correct an incorrect response. Give no assistance.

TEACHING PROCEDURE

STEP 1: Use oversize sock, beginning with the cuff of oversize sock pushed down to the resident's right ankle. The trainer assists the resident to hold cuff of the sock, placing the resident's thumbs inside and fingers outside, and says, "JOHN, PUT ON YOUR SOCK", and immediately assists the resident to pull the cuff of his sock from his ankle to the calf of his leg.

STEP 2: Use oversize sock. Begin with the cuff of oversize sock pushed down to the resident's right ankle. The trainer assists resident to hold cuff of the sock, placing the resident's thumbs inside and fingers outside, and say, "JOHN, PUT ON YOUR SOCK", and immediately assists the resident to pull the cuff of his sock from his ankle to the calf of his leg.

STEP 3: Use oversized sock. Begin with cuff or oversized sock slightly below the right heel and say, "JOHN, PUT ON YOUR SOCK", and immediately assists the resident to pull cuff of the sock up and over the calf of leg.

STEP 4: Use oversize sock. Begin with cuff of oversized sock at mid-arch of right foot and say, "JOHN, PUT ON YOUR SOCK", and immediately assists resident to pull cuff of sock up and over heel to full leg.

STEP 5: Use oversize sock. Place oversize sock beside the resident's right foot. The trainer assists the resident to align sock with front of foot and place thumb inside and fingers outside of cuffs, and says, "JOHN, PUT ON YOUR SOCK", and immediately assists the resident to pull cuff of sock up and over to the calf of leg.

STEP 6: Use oversize sock. Place oversize sock beside the resident's right foot. The trainer assists the resident to align sock with front of foot and place thumb inside and fingers outside of cuffs, and says, "JOHN, PUT ON YOUR SOCK", and immediately assists the resident to put sock over toes and pull sock to calf of leg. (See note 1).

STEP 7: Terminal Behavior. Use normal size sock. Place fitted sock beside the resident's right foot. The trainer touches sock and says, "JOHN, PUT ON YOUR SOCK". Give minimal reinforcement and assistance as required. (See note 2).

NOTE 1: If the resident is having difficulty with correct positioning of sock, e.g., confusing the heel with the toe part, a sock marked with colors (toe - red, heel - blue) may be used. In order to teach correct toe-nail position, trainer may color the resident's toe red and heel blue to match the sock. Then the resident may be shown how to align the sock using these color prompts. This prompting should be gradually faded out until criterion is reached with the unmarked sock.

NOTE 2: If the resident has difficulty with the normal size sock, try putting talcum powder or corn starch in the sock, and on the resident's foot to help alleviate the difficulty of the foot resisting as it is pushed into the sock.

MODEL LESSON 004
TASK: TAKING OFF SOCK.

GOAL: Improve dressing skills.

OBJECTIVE: To teach the resident to take off his sock upon request.

MATERIALS: Nylon stretch sock two sizes too large for the resident; a nylon stretch sock resident's normal size.

SETTING: Resident and trainer sitting on the floor, resident with shoes and socks off.

PRE-TEST/POST-TEST: Use normal size sock. Begin with one sock completely on the resident's right foot. The trainer touches sock and says, "JOHN, TAKE OFF YOUR SOCK". Do not reinforce a correct response. And, do not correct an incorrect response. Give no assistance.

TEACHING PROCEDURE

STEP 1: Use oversize sock. Begin with cuff of oversize sock at mid-arch of the resident's right foot. The trainer assists the resident to hold cuff of sock, placing the resident's thumbs inside and fingers outside, and says, "JOHN, TAKE OFF YOUR SOCK", and immediately assists the resident to push the sock clear of his foot.

STEP 2: Use oversize sock. Begin with cuff of oversize sock slightly below right heel. The trainer assists the resident to hold cuff of sock and says, "JOHN, TAKE OFF YOUR SOCK", and immediately assists the resident to push the sock clear of foot.

STEP 3: Use oversize sock. Begin with cuff of oversize sock at right ankle (above heel), and say, "JOHN, TAKE OFF YOUR SOCK", and immediately assist the resident to push sock past heel and clear of foot.

STEP 4: Use oversize sock. Begin with oversize sock completely on the resident's right foot and say, "JOHN, TAKE OFF YOUR SOCK", and immediately assist the resident to push sock past ankle, heel and clear the foot.

STEP 5: Terminal behavior. Use normal size sock. Begin with fitted sock completely on the resident's right foot. The trainer touches sock and says, "JOHN, TAKE OFF YOUR SOCK". (See note 1).

NOTE 1. If the resident has difficulty with the normal sized sock, try putting talcum powder or corn starch in the sock and on the resident's foot to help alleviate the difficulty of the foot resisting as it is pulled out of the sock.

MODEL LESSON 005
TASK: PUTTING ON T-SHIRT (PULLOVER TYPE).

GOAL: Improve dressing skills.

OBJECTIVE: To teach the resident to put on his shirt upon request, without discriminating front from back.

MATERIALS: A t-shirt two sizes too large for the resident, and a normal size t-shirt for the resident. (The t-shirts should be the cotton type, with loose fitting neck and short sleeves).

SETTING: The resident sits, the trainer stands near resident. The resident is bare-chested.

PRE-TEST/POST-TEST: (Use normal size t-shirt): Begin with shirt placed flat and front-down on the resident's lap. The trainer touches shirt saying, "JOHN, PUT ON YOUR T-SHIRT". Do not reinforce a correct response and do not correct an incorrect response. Give no assistance.

TEACHING PROCEDURE

STEP 1: Use over-size t-shirt in steps 1 through 4. Begin with oversize t-shirt on the resident. The trainer raises the resident's arms and lifts neck hole up and over the resident's head so that the body of the shirt is covering the resident's head and the resident's arms are extended upward but still in the sleeves. The trainer says, "JOHN, PUT ON YOUR T-SHIRT", and immediately assists the resident to look through the neck hole and lift up and push back his arms so that his head will automatically be pushed through the neck hole. The shirt will then fall down to the resident's waist, if not, the resident can be assisted to position the t-shirt properly.

STEP 2: Use over-size t-shirt. Begin with oversize t-shirt off the resident. The trainer puts t-shirt partially on the resident so that the shoulder holes are at resident's mid-arm and the back of the t-shirt is gathered at the resident's shoulders. The trainer then says, "JOHN, PUT ON YOUR T-SHIRT", and immediately assists the resident to lift up the gathered back of his t-shirt and pull the t-shirt over his head until he can look through the neck hole. The resident should then complete action to position the t-shirt properly.

STEP 3: Demonstration: Begin with oversize t-shirt off the resident. The trainer puts the t-shirt partially on the resident so that the shoulder holes are at the resident's wrist and body of the t-shirt surrounds extended arms. The trainer says, "JOHN, PUT ON YOUR T-SHIRT", and immediately assists the resident to grasp the right side of resident's t-shirt with his left hand and pull the t-shirt with his left hand and pull the t-shirt until the shoulder hole is at mid-arm. Repeat similar action with the left side of the t-shirt. The resident should then complete action to position the t-shirt properly. (See note 1).

STEP 4: Use oversize t-shirt. Begin with oversize t-shirt placed flat and front-down on the resident's lap. Trainer says, "JOHN, PUT ON YOUR T-SHIRT", and immediately assists the resident to lift up the back of his t-shirt, and put his right hand through the right shoulder hole and his left hand through the left shoulder hole so that the shoulder holes are at the resident's wrists. The resident should then complete the action to position the t-shirt properly.

STEP 5: Terminal Behavior. (Use normal size t-shirt). Begin with fitted t-shirt placed flat and front down on the resident's lap. The trainer then touches the t-shirt and says, "JOHN, PUT ON YOUR T-SHIRT". Give minimal reinforcement and assistance as required.

NOTE 1: The trainer may wish to teach the resident to put on his t-shirt using another method. If another approach seems easier for the resident, the trainer should make the appropriate revisions in the teaching procedure. One alternative teaching method would be to allow the resident to raise his arms so that the t-shirt will fall from the resident's wrists to his mid-arms. (Whether this works or not may depend upon the t-shirt's material and the width of the shoulder holes. Use whatever teaching method that works most easily with the resident.)

MODEL LESSON 006
TASK: TAKING OFF T-SHIRT (PULLOVER TYPE)

GOAL: Improve dressing skills.

OBJECTIVE: To teach the resident to take off his t-shirt upon request.

MATERIALS: A t-shirt two sizes too large for the resident; a t-shirt of resident's normal size. (T-shirts should be the cotton pullover type, with loose fitting neck and short sleeves).

SETTING: The resident sits, the trainer stands near the resident.

PRE-TEST/POST-TEST: Use normal-size t-shirt. Begin with t-shirt and says, "JOHN, TAKE OFF YOUR T-SHIRT". Do not reinforce a correct response and do not correct an incorrect response. Give no assistance.

TEACHING PROCEDURE

STEP 1: Use oversize t-shirt in steps 1 through 3. Begin with over size t-shirt on the resident. The trainer grasps the bottom of the resident's t-shirt by the sides, pulls the t-shirt inside out and up over the resident's chest and head until the shirt is only covering the resident's extended arms and hands. The trainer says, "JOHN, TAKE OFF YOUR T-SHIRT", and immediately assists the resident to grasp the left side of the resident's shirt with his right hand and pull his left arm and hand clear of the t-shirt. Repeat similar action with right side of the t-shirt, completely removing the resident's t-shirt. (See note 1).

STEP 2: Use oversize t-shirt. Begin with oversize t-shirt on the resident. The trainer grasps the bottom of the resident's t-shirt by the sides, pulls the t-shirt inside-out and up over the resident's chest until the t-shirt is covering the resident's head and resident's arms are extended over his head. The trainer says, "JOHN, TAKE OFF YOUR T-SHIRT," and immediately assists the resident to grasp the left side of the resident's t-shirt with his right hand

and pull his t-shirt over his head and free of arm and hand, and, then, assists the resident to remove the right side of his t-shirt.

STEP 3: Use oversized shirt. Begin with oversized shirt completely on the resident. The trainer says, "JOHN, TAKE OFF YOUR T-SHIRT", and immediately assists the resident to grasp the right side of his t-shirt with his left hand and the left side of his t-shirt with his right. Then, assist the resident to pull the t-shirt up until the inside-out t-shirt is covering the resident's head and resident's arms are extended over his head. The resident should then complete action to remove his t-shirt properly.

STEP 4: Terminal behavior. Use normal sized t-shirt. Begin with fitted t-shirt completely on the resident. The trainer touches the t-shirt and says, "JOHN, TAKE OFF YOUR T-SHIRT". Give minimal reinforcement and assistance as required.

NOTE 1. The trainer may wish to teach the resident to take off his t-shirt using another method. If another approach seems easier for the resident, the trainer should make the appropriate revisions in the teaching procedure. One alternative teaching method would be to allow the resident to lower his arms so that the t-shirt will fall to the resident's wrists then drop to the floor. (Whether this works or not may depend upon the t-shirt's material and the width of the shoulder holes). Use whatever teaching method that works most easily with the resident.

MODEL LESSON 007
TASK: PUTTING ON PANTS.

GOAL: Improve dressing skills.

OBJECTIVE: To teach the resident to put on his pants upon request, without zipping, snapping, or discriminating front from back.

MATERIALS: A pair of pants two sizes too large for the resident; a pair of pants the resident's size. Both have elastic waistbands.

SETTING: As indicated by each step. (See note 1).

PRE-TEST/POST-TEST: Use normal sized pants. The resident is sitting on the edge of a chair. Give the resident his pants. The trainer touches the pants and says, "JOHN, PUT ON YOUR PANTS". Do not reinforce a correct response and do not correct an incorrect response.

TEACHING PROCEDURE

STEP 1: DEMONSTRATION - Use oversize pants in steps 1 through 5. The resident is standing. Begin with oversize pants at the resident's mid-hip level. The trainer says: "JOHN, PUT ON YOUR PANTS", and immediately assists the resident to grasp the waistband (his thumbs hooked over the waistband and his fingers outside, pulling upward) and pull his pants up to the waist level.

STEP 2: Use oversize pants. The resident is standing. Begin with over-size pants at the resident's knee level. The trainer says, "JOHN, PUT ON YOUR PANTS", and immediately assists the resident to grasp the waistband (thumbs hooked over the waistband, fingers outside) and pull pants up from knees to waist level.

STEP 3: Use oversize pants. The resident is standing. Begin with oversize pants pushed down to the resident's feet, with feet still showing. The trainer says, "JOHN, PUT ON YOUR PANTS", and immediately assists the resident to grasp the waistband and pull pants up from feet to waist level.

STEP 4: Use oversize pants. The resident is sitting on the edge of a chair. Put the resident's feet into leg holes so that the waistband is at the resident's ankles and pants legs are stretched out. The trainer says, "JOHN, PUT ON YOUR PANTS", and immediately assists the resident to pick up his right foot and pull up the sides of the right pants leg until his feet are visible. The trainer assists the resident to place his foot on the floor. Repeat similar action with the left foot. The resident should then stand up and pull pants up from his feet to his waist level.

STEP 5: Use oversized pants. The resident is sitting on the edge of a chair. Give the resident his pants. The trainer says, "JOHN, PUT ON YOUR PANTS", and immediately assists the resident to grasp waistband (so that leg holes are visible and positioned across from the appropriate legs) and put each leg in the appropriate leg hole. The resident should then complete action until the pants are pulled to waist level.

STEP 6: Terminal behavior: Use normal sized pants. The resident is sitting on the edge of a chair. Give the resident his pants. The trainer touches pants and says, "JOHN, PUT ON YOUR PANTS". Give minimal reinforcement and assistance as required.

MODEL LESSON 008
TASK: TAKING OFF PANTS.

GOAL: Improve dressing skills.

OBJECTIVE: To teach the resident to take off his pants upon request, without unsnapping or unzipping.

MATERIALS: A pair of pants two sizes too large for the resident, and a pair of pants the resident's normal size. Both have elastic waistbands.

SETTING: As indicated by each step. (See note 1).

PRE-TEST/POST-TEST: Use normal sized pants. The resident is standing near a chair. Begin with pants completely on the resident. The trainer touches the pants and says, "JOHN, TAKE OFF YOUR PANTS". Do not reinforce a correct response and do not correct an incorrect response. Give no assistance.

TEACHING PROCEDURE

STEP 1: Use oversized pants in step 1 through 3. The resident is sitting on the edge of a chair. Begin with oversized pants pushed down so that the waistband is at the resident's feet. The trainer says, "JOHN, TAKE OFF YOUR PANTS", and immediately assists the resident to lift his right leg and bend his knee so the resident can grasp the right pants cuff and pull the pants leg up and clear of the resident's foot. Repeat similar action with left leg.

STEP 2: Use oversized pants. The resident is standing near a chair. Begin with waistband of oversized pants just above the resident's knees. The trainer says, "JOHN, TAKE OFF YOUR PANTS", and immediately assists the resident to grasp the waistband at both sides (thumbs hooked over waistband, fingers outside and pushing downward) and push pants down so that the waistband is at the resident's feet. The resident should then sit down on the edge of a chair and complete action to remove pants.

STEP 3: Use oversized pants. The resident is standing near a chair. Begin with waistband of oversized pants at the resident's waist level. The trainer says, "JOHN, TAKE OFF YOUR PANTS", and immediately assists the resident to grasp the waistband, fingers outside and push pants down so that the waistband is at the resident's feet. The resident should then sit down on the edge of a chair and complete action to remove pants.

STEP 4: Terminal behavior: Use normal sized pants. The resident is standing near a chair. Begin with fitted pants completely on the resident. The trainer touches the pants and says, "JOHN, TAKE OFF YOUR PANTS". Give minimal reinforcement and assistance as required.

NOTE 1: This lesson plan allows the resident to sit while performing certain sub-skills, in order to facilitate learning.

MODEL LESSON 009
TASK: PUTTING ON DRESS.

GOAL: Improve dressing skills.

OBJECTIVE: To teach the resident to put on her dress upon request, without buttoning or zipping.

MATERIALS: A dress two sizes too large for the resident, and a dress the resident's normal size. Both open at the back, have short sleeves, and are unbuttoned and unzipped.

SETTING: The resident and the trainer standing beside the table or bed.

PRE-TEST/POST-TEST: Use normal sized dress. Give the resident her dress. The trainer touches the dress and says, "JANE, PUT ON YOUR DRESS". Do not reinforce a correct response. Give no assistance.

TEACHING PROCEDURE

STEP 1: Use oversize dress in steps 1 through 5. Begin with shoulders of oversize dress at the resident's elbow and bodice of dress down at resident's waist. The trainer says, "JANE, PUT ON YOUR DRESS", and immediately assists the resident to grasp the right shoulder of her dress with her left hand, pull the dress up to the resident's shoulder and position it properly. Repeat similar action with left shoulder of dress.

STEP 2: Begin with the resident's arms out of arm holes and bodice of oversized dress at the resident's waist, the trainer says, "JANE, PUT ON YOUR DRESS", and immediately assists the resident to grasp right shoulder of dress with left hand so that right arm hole is visible, put right arm into arm hole and pull shoulder of dress up to the resident's shoulder and position it properly. Repeat similar action with left shoulder of dress.

STEP 3: Place the resident's oversized dress front down on a table or bed. The trainer lifts up back of dress. The trainer says, "JANE, PUT ON YOUR DRESS," and immediately assists the resident to bend down, inserting her arms and head through the opening, and straighten up, so that the bodice of dress falls down to the resident's waist. The resident should then complete action to position dress properly.

STEP 4: Place the resident's oversize dress front down on a table or bed. The trainer says, "JANE, PUT ON YOUR DRESS", and immediately assists the resident to lift up back of dress, bend down and insert arms and head through the opening, and straighten up so that the bodice of dress falls down to the resident's waist. The resident should then complete action to position dress properly.

STEP 5: Give the resident her oversize dress. The trainer says, "JANE, PUT ON YOUR DRESS", and immediately assists the resident to place dress front down on a bed or table. The resident should then complete action to position dress properly.

STEP 6: Terminal Behavior. Use normal size dress. Give the resident her dress. The trainer touches dress and says, "JANE, PUT ON YOUR DRESS". Give minimal reinforcement and assistance as required.

MODEL LESSON 010
TASK: TAKING OFF DRESS.

GOAL: Improve dressing skills.

OBJECTIVE: To teach the resident to take off her dress upon request without unbuttoning or unzipping.

MATERIALS: A dress two sizes too large for the resident; a dress the resident's normal size. Both open at the back, have short sleeves, and are unbuttoned or unzipped.

SETTING: The resident and trainer stand, facing each other.

PRE-TEST/POST-TEST: Use normal size dress. Begin with dress completely on the resident. The trainer touches the dress and says, "JANE, TAKE OFF YOUR DRESS".

TEACHING PROCEDURE

STEP 1: Use oversize dress in steps through 3. Begin with the resident's arms out of arm holes and bodice of oversize dress down around the resident's waist. The trainer says, "JANE, TAKE OFF YOUR DRESS", and immediately assists the resident to grasp the waistline of her dress at the sides, push it down to her feet, and step clear of the dress.

STEP 2: Use oversize dress. Begin with shoulders of oversized dress at the resident's elbows and bodice of dress around the resident's waist. The trainer says. "JANE, TAKE OFF YOUR DRESS", and immediately assist the resident to grasp right shoulder of dress with left hand and pull right arm out of arm hole. Repeat similar action with left shoulder of dress. The resident should then complete action to remove her dress.

STEP 3: Use oversize dress. Begin with the resident's oversize dress completely on. The trainer says, "JANE, TAKE OFF YOUR DRESS", and immediately assists the resident to grasp right shoulder of dress with left hand and pull shoulder to the resident's right elbow. The resident should pull right arm out of arm hole. Repeat similar action with other side of dress. The resident should then complete action to remove her dress.

STEP 4: Terminal behavior. Use normal size dress. Begin with normal size dress completely on the resident. The trainer touches dress and says, "JANE, TAKE OFF YOUR DRESS". Give minimal reinforcement and assistance as required.

MODEL LESSON 011
TASK: PUTTING ON COAT.

GOAL: Improve dressing skills.

OBJECTIVE: To teach the resident to put on his coat upon request, without buttoning or zipping.

MATERIALS: A coat two sizes too large for the resident; a coat the resident's normal size. Both are unbuttoned and unzipped.

SETTING: The resident and trainer standing, facing each other.

PRE-TEST/POST TEST: Use normal size coat. Give the resident his coat. The trainer touches the coat and says, "JOHN, PUT ON YOUR COAT". Do not reinforce a correct response and do not correct an incorrect response. Give no assistance.

TEACHING PROCEDURE

STEP 1: Use oversize coat in steps 1 through 2. Begin with the shoulder of coat slightly below the resident's shoulders. The trainer says, "JOHN, PUT ON YOUR COAT", and immediately assists the resident to raise his arms to the shoulder level with an exaggerated forceful movement, causing his coat to be lifted to the shoulder level. The trainer then assists the resident to grasp the right lapel with his right hand and the left lapel with his left hand and to position his coat properly on his shoulders. (See Note 1).

STEP 2: Use oversize coat. Begin with shoulders of oversize coat at the resident's elbows. The trainer says, "JOHN, PUT ON YOUR COAT", and immediately assists the resident to complete action to position coat properly.

MODEL LESSON 012
TASK: TAKING OFF COAT.

GOAL: Improve dressing skills.

OBJECTIVE: To teach the resident to take off his coat upon request, without unbuttoning or unzipping.

MATERIALS: A coat two sizes too large for the resident, and a coat the resident's normal size. Both are unbuttoned and unzipped.

SETTING: The resident and trainer standing, facing each other.

PRE-TEST/POST-TEST: Use normal size coat. Begin with the coat completely on the resident. The trainer touches the coat and says, "JOHN, TAKE OFF YOUR COAT". Do not reinforce a correct response and do not correct an incorrect response. Give no assistance.

TEACHING PROCEDURE

STEP 1: Use oversize coat in steps 1 through 2. Begin with coat shoulders at the resident's elbows, and body of coat hanging loosely behind him. The trainer says, "JOHN, TAKE OFF YOUR COAT", and immediately assists the resident to reach across the front of his body with his left hand, grasp the right sleeve at the wrist and pull sleeve clear of resident's arm. Repeat similar action with left sleeve, and completely remove the resident's coat.

STEP 2: Use oversize coat. Begin with oversize coat completely on the resident. The trainer says, "JOHN, TAKE OFF YOUR COAT", and immediately assist the resident to grasp right side of coat at waist level with right hand and left side with left hand and push coat off the resident's shoulders so that the shoulders of coat are at the resident's elbows. The resident should then complete action to remove the resident's coat.

STEP 3: Terminal Behavior. Use normal size coat. Begin with normal size coat completely on the resident. The trainer touches the coat and says, "JOHN, TAKE OFF YOUR COAT". Give minimal reinforcement and assistance as required.

MODEL LESSON 013
TASK: PUTTING ON SHIRT (BUTTON-DOWN).

GOAL: Improve dressing skills.

OBJECTIVE: To teach the resident to put on his shirt upon request, without buttoning or zipping.

MATERIALS: A shirt two sizes too large for the resident, a shirt the resident's normal size. Both are unbuttoned and unzipped.

SETTING: The resident and trainer standing, facing each other.

PRE-TEST/ POST-TEST: Use normal size shirt. Give the resident his shirt. The trainer touches and says, "JOHN, PUT ON YOUR SHIRT". Do not correct an incorrect response. Give no assistance.

TEACHING PROCEDURE

STEP 1: Use oversize shirt in steps 1 through 5. Begin with shoulders of shirt slightly below the residents shoulders. The trainer says, "JOHN, PUT ON YOUR SHIRT", and immediately assists the resident to raise his arms to the shoulder level with an exaggerated forceful movement, causing his shirt to be lifted to the shoulder level. The trainer then assists the resident to grasp the right lapel with his left hand to position his shirt properly on his shoulders.

STEP 2: Use oversize shirt. Begin with shoulders of oversize shirt at the residents elbow. The trainer says, "JOHN, PUT ON YOUR SHIRT", and immediately assists the resident to complete action to position his shirt properly.

STEP 3: Use oversize shirt. Begin with the resident's left arm in left shirt sleeve and the resident's right arm out of right sleeves. The trainer positions right arm hole near resident's right elbow. The trainer says, "JOHN, PUT ON YOUR SHIRT", and immediately assists the resident to insert right arm into sleeve so that shoulder of shirt is at the resident's right elbow. The resident should then complete action to position properly.

STEP 4: Use oversize shirt. Begin with the resident's left arm in left shirt sleeve and resident's right arm out of right sleeve. The trainer says, "JOHN, PUT ON YOUR SHIRT", and immediately assists the resident to reach for and locate right arm hole and insert his arm into sleeve so that shoulder of shirt is at the resident's right elbow. The resident should then complete action to position properly.

STEP 5: Use oversize shirt. Give the resident his shirt. The trainer says, "JOHN, PUT ON YOUR SHIRT", and immediately assists the resident to grasp right shoulder of shirt with left hand so that right arm hole is visible, and push right arm into arm hole until shoulder of shirt is at resident's right elbow. The resident should then complete action to position properly.

STEP 6: Terminal Behavior. Use normal size shirt. Give the resident his shirt. The trainer touches shirt and says, "JOHN, PUT ON YOUR SHIRT". Give minimal reinforcement and assistance as required.

NOTE 1: The trainer may wish to teach the resident to put on his shirt/coat using another method. If another approach seems easier for the resident the trainer should make the appropriate revisions in the Teaching Procedure used for that resident. One alternative would be is to have the resident put his shirt/coat on a table or bed so that it is open (with the lapels turned back and the lining visible) and it is positioned upside-down. The resident would then put each arm in the appropriate arm hole and flip the shirt/coat up over his head, pushing his arms through the sleeves. The resident would then position the shirt/coat properly on his shoulders and button, starting at bottom of shirt and buttoning upward. If the resident, however, has difficulties with the normal size shirt/coat, try having the resident wear a light weight short-sleeved shirt rather than a heavy long-sleeved shirt to help alleviate the difficulty of the shirt/coat resisting as the arm is pushed into the shirt/coat sleeve.

MODEL LESSON 014
TASK: TAKING OFF SHIRT (BUTTON-DOWN).

GOAL: Improve dressing skills.

OBJECTIVE: To teach the resident to take off his unbuttoned shirt upon request.

MATERIALS: A shirt two sizes too large for the resident; a shirt of resident's normal size, both being unbuttoned.

SETTING: The resident and trainer are standing, facing each other.

PRE-TEST/POST-TEST: Use normal size shirt. Begin with shirt completely on the resident. The trainer touches and says, "JOHN, TAKE OFF YOUR SHIRT". Do not reinforce a correct response and do not correct an incorrect response. Give no assistance.

TEACHING PROCEDURE

STEP 1: Use oversize shirt in steps 1 through 2. Begin with shirt shoulders at the resident's elbows, and body of shirt hanging loosely behind him. The trainer says, "JOHN, TAKE OFF YOUR SHIRT", and immediately assists the resident to reach across the front of his body with his left hand, grasp the right sleeve at the wrist and pull sleeve clear of the resident's arm. Repeat similar action with left sleeve, completely removing the resident's shirt.

STEP 2: Use oversize shirt. Begin with oversize shirt completely on the resident. The trainer says, "JOHN, TAKE OFF YOUR SHIRT", and immediately assists the resident to grasp right side of shirt at waist level with right hand and left side with left hand and push shirt off resident's shoulders so that the shoulders of shirt are at the resident's elbows. The resident should then complete action to remove the resident's shirt.

STEP 3: Terminal Behavior. Use normal size shirt. Begin with normal size shirt completely on the resident. The trainer touches the shirt and says, "JOHN, TAKE OFF YOUR SHIRT". Give minimal reinforcement and assistance as required.

MODEL LESSON 015
TASK: PUTTING ON SHOES.

GOAL: Improve dressing skills.

OBJECTIVE: To teach the resident to put on his shoe upon request, without discriminating the right shoe from the left shoe and without lacing.

MATERIALS: A moccasin - type right shoe or right loafer two sizes too large for the resident; a tie - type right shoe the resident's normal size. Both have laces removed or loosened. (A shoehorn is optional).

SETTING: The resident and trainer sitting on floor, resident with socks on and shoes off.

PRE-TEST/ POST-TEST: Use normal size shoe. Place right shoe besides the resident's right foot. The trainer touches shoe and says, "JOHN, PUT ON YOUR SHOE". Do not reinforce a correct response and do not correct an incorrect response. Give no assistance.

TEACHING PROCEDURE

STEP 1: Use oversize loafer-type shoe. Begin with the resident's right heel half-way inside the oversize shoe. The trainer assists the resident to hold shoe tongue (or top of shoe) up with one hand and to place shoe horn (or index finger of other hand) down inside the back of the shoe. The trainer says. "JOHN, PUT ON YOUR SHOE", and immediately assists the resident to push his heel into the shoe.

STEP 2: Use oversize shoe. Begin with the resident's right heel outside the oversize shoe, toes inside. The trainer assists the resident to hold shoe tongue (or top of shoe) and to use shoehorn or index finger. The trainer says, "JOHN, PUT ON YOUR SHOE", and immediately assists the resident to push heel into shoe.

STEP 3: Use oversize shoe. Place oversize right shoe beside the resident's right foot. The trainer assists resident to align shoe with front of foot, hold shoe tongue (or top of shoe) and use shoehorn (or index finger). The trainer says, "JOHN, PUT ON YOUR SHOE", and immediately assists the resident to put toes into shoe and push heel into shoe.

STEP 4: Terminal Behavior. Use normal size loafer or tie-type shoe. Place fitted right shoe beside the resident's right foot. The trainer touches shoe and says, "JOHN, PUT ON YOUR SHOE". (See Note 1).

NOTE 1: If the resident has difficulty with the normal-size shoe, try putting talcum powder or corn starch on the bottom of sock and inside the resident's shoe to help alleviate the difficulty of the sock resisting as it is pushed into the shoe. Once the resident has mastered tying and right - left shoe discrimination, those tasks may also be required as part of the resident's putting on his shoes.

MODEL LESSON 016
TASK: TAKING OFF SHOE

GOAL: Improve dressing skills.

OBJECTIVE: To teach the resident to take off his shoe upon request.

MATERIALS: A moccasin - type right shoe or right loafer two sizes too large for the resident; a tie-type right shoe the resident's normal size. Both have laces removed or loosened.

SETTING: The resident and trainer sitting on the floor, resident with sock on and shoes off.

PRE-TEST/POST-TEST: Use normal size tie-type shoe. Begin with right shoe completely on the resident's right foot. The trainer touches the shoe and says, "JOHN, TAKE OFF YOUR SHOE". Do not reinforce a correct response and do not correct an incorrect response. Give no assistance.

TEACHING PROCEDURE

STEP 1: Demonstration - Use oversize loafer-type shoe. Begin with the resident's right heel outside shoe, toes inside. The trainer assists the resident to hold heel of oversize shoe and say, "JOHN, TAKE OFF YOUR SHOE", and immediately assists the resident to push the shoe clear of his foot.

STEP 2: Use oversize loafer. Begin with the resident's right heel half-way outside the shoe. The trainer assists the resident to hold heel of the shoe and says, "JOHN, TAKE OFF YOUR SHOE", and immediately assists the resident to pull the heel out of the shoe until the shoe is clear of the foot.

STEP 3: Use oversize loafer. Begin with oversize right shoe completely on the resident's right foot. The trainer says, "JOHN, TAKE OFF YOUR SHOE", and immediately assists the resident to push the shoe clear of foot.

STEP 4: Terminal Behavior. Use normal size loafer or tie-type shoe. Begin with fitted right shoe completely on the resident's right foot. The trainer touches the shoe and says, "JOHN, TAKE OFF YOUR SHOE".

Note 1: If the resident has difficulty with the normal-size shoe, try putting talcum powder or corn starch on the bottom of the sock and inside the resident's shoe to help alleviate the difficulty of the sock resisting as it is pulled out of the shoe. Once the resident has mastered untying, this task may also be required as part of the resident's taking off his shoe.

MODEL LESSON 017
TASK: ZIPPING JACKET

GOAL: Improve dressing skills.

OBJECTIVE: To teach the resident to zip a zipper upon request.

MATERIALS: A jacket with a large zipper (½ inch wide); a jacket with normal size zipper (¼ inch wide).

SETTING: The resident and trainer standing, facing each other.

PRE-TEST/POST-TEST: Put the jacket with normal size zipper on the resident. Begin with the resident's jacket completely unzipped. The trainer touches the zipper and says, "JOHN, ZIP UP YOUR JACKET". Do not reinforce a correct response and do not correct an incorrect response. Give no assistance.

TEACHING PROCEDURE

STEP 1: Put the jacket with a large zipper on the resident in steps 1 through 4. Begin with the large zipper tab pulled half way to zipper top. The trainer says, "JOHN, ZIP UP YOUR JACKET", and immediately assists the resident to push the tab down flat against the zipper so that the catch is locked.

STEP 2: Use large zipper. Begin with the large zipper tab pulled to, but not off, the zipper and the trainer says, "JOHN, ZIP UP YOUR JACKET", and immediately assists the resident to hold the zipper and with his left hand, and pull the zipper top, and push tab down flat against the zipper.

STEP 3: Use large zipper. Begin with the resident's jacket completely unzipped. The trainer pulls opposite sides of the jacket together and aligns the zipper tab with the zipper and, the trainer says, "JOHN, ZIP UP YOUR JACKET", and immediately assists the resident to insert the zipper and into the zipper tab. The resident should then complete action to finish zipping.

STEP 4: Use large zipper. Begin with the resident's jacket completely unzipped. The trainer says, "JOHN, ZIP UP YOUR JACKET", and immediately assists the resident to pull opposite sides of the jacket together and to align the zipper tab with the zipper end. The resident should then insert the zipper end into the zipper tab and complete action to finish zipping.

STEP 5: Terminal Behavior. Put the jacket with normal size zipper on the resident. Begin with the resident's jacket completely unzipped. The trainer touches the zipper and says, "JOHN, ZIP UP YOUR JACKET". Give minimal reinforcement and assistance as required.

NOTE: If the resident has difficulty with this task or with subsequent zipping tasks, the trainer should stop work on the step and initiate practice on more basic skills needed for zipping. The trainer might have the resident practice merely picking up and manipulating the zipper tab (a prerequisite needed in step 1), and making vertical sweeping gestures with his wrist (a prerequisite skill needed in step 3). Then, if such practice is not sufficient to alleviate the difficulty in this step, the trainer might have the resident do each step of lesson plan using a "zipper board" that is first placed on a table in front of the resident. (This will enable the resident to work away from his body and to see more clearly what he is doing). Give the resident steps 1 through 3 using this method; and then after the resident has mastered this task, go back and re-do those steps using the "zipper board" placed against the resident's stomach. (This will enable the resident to work near his body, approximating the terminal behavior). Then after the resident has mastered this, go back and re-do steps 1 through 3 using a jacket on the resident.

MODEL LESSON 018
TASK: UNZIPPING JACKET

GOAL: Improve dressing skills.

OBJECTIVE: To teach the resident how to unzip the zipper on his jacket upon request.

MATERIALS: A jacket with a large zipper (½ inch wide); a jacket with a normal size zipper (¼ inch wide).

SETTING: The resident and trainer standing, facing each other.

PRE-TEST/POST-TEST: Put the jacket with normal size zipper on the resident. Begin with the resident's jacket fully zipped. The trainer touches the zipper and says, "JOHN, UNZIP YOUR JACKET". Do not reinforce a correct response and do not correct an incorrect response. Give no assistance.

TEACHING PROCEDURE

STEP 1: Put jacket with a large zipper on the resident in steps 1 through 3. Begin with a large zipper tab pulled to, but not off the zipper and the trainer says, "JOHN, UNZIP YOUR JACKET", and immediately assist the resident to pull the zipper tab up and out so that the catch is released and to pull the tab off the zipper end.

STEP 2: Use large zipper. Begin with the large zipper tab pulled half way to zipper end. The trainer says, "JOHN, UNZIP YOUR JACKET", and immediately assists the resident to pull the zipper tab up and out to pull the tab down and off the zipper end.

STEP 3: Use large zipper. Begin with the large zipper pulled all the way up. The trainer says, "JOHN, UNZIP YOUR JACKET", and immediately assists the resident to pull zipper tab up and out and to pull tab down and off zipper end.

STEP 4: Terminal Behavior. Put jacket with normal sized zipper on the resident. Begin with the resident's jacket fully zipped. The trainer touches the zipper and says, "JOHN, UNZIP YOUR JACKET". Give minimal reinforcement and assistance as required.

NOTE: If the resident has difficulty with this task or with the subsequent unzipping tasks, the trainer should stop work on the step and initiate practice on the more basic skills needed for zipping. The trainer might have the resident practice merely picking up and manipulating the zipper tab and making vertical sweeping gestures with his wrist, then if such practice is not sufficient to alleviate the difficulty in the problem step. The trainer might have the resident to do each step of the lesson plan again using a "zipper board" that is first placed on a table in front of the resident. Give the resident steps 1 through 3 using this frame; then after the resident has mastered this, go back and re-do those steps using the zipper board placed flat against the resident's stomach. Then after the resident has mastered this, go back and re-do steps 1 through 3 using a jacket on the resident.

MODEL LESSON 019
TASK: BUTTONING SHIRT

GOAL: Improve dressing skills.

OBJECTIVE: To teach the resident to button his shirt upon request.

MATERIALS: A shirt or vest with large buttons (½ inch or larger) and buttonholes (½ inch larger) than the buttons; A shirt or vest with normal size buttons and buttonholes.

SETTING: The resident and trainer sitting facing each other.

PRE-TEST/POST-TEST: (Put shirt or vest with normal size buttonholes on the resident.) Begin with the resident's shirt completely unbuttoned. The trainer says, "JOHN, BUTTON YOUR SHIRT". Do not reinforce a correct response and do not correct an incorrect response.

TEACHING PROCEDURE

STEP 1: Put the shirt or vest with large buttonholes on the resident in steps 1 through 4. Begin with bottom button pushed half way into buttonhole. The trainer says, "JOHN, BUTTON YOUR SHIRT", and immediately assists the resident to (a) grasp the left edge of button with his left thumb and forefinger and to (b) grasp the right edge of that buttonhole over and then under the button. Repeat demonstration with the remainder of the buttons, beginning at the bottom and working up. The trainer repeats command each time with each button.

STEP 2: Use large buttons and buttonholes. Begin with shirt or vest completely unbuttoned. The trainer aligns the bottom button with the bottom buttonhole. The trainer places the resident's left hand so that the thumb is over the buttonhole and the forefinger is on the back side of the cloth. The trainer turns the left side of the edge of the shirt perpendicular to the resident's body. The trainer touches the bottom button and says, "JOHN, BUTTON YOUR SHIRT", and immediately assists the resident to grasp the right edge of the button with the right thumb and forefinger and push the button through the buttonhole and against the left thumb. The trainer should then assist the resident to (a) release the left forefinger from the backside of the cloth and, (b) replace it on the right edge of the buttonhole. The resident should then complete action or buttoning. Repeat the demonstration with the remainder of the buttons, beginning at the bottom and working up.

STEP 3: Use large buttons and buttonholes. Begin with a shirt or vest completely unbuttoned. The trainer aligns the bottom button with bottom buttonhole. The trainer touches bottom button and says, "JOHN, BUTTON YOUR SHIRT", and immediately assists the resident to grasp buttonhole with his left hand so that the thumb is over the hole and the forefinger is on the backside of the cloth and to turn left side of the shirt edge perpendicular to the resident's body. The resident should then complete action of buttoning. Repeat demonstration with the remainder of the buttons, beginning at the bottom and working up.

STEP 4: Use large buttons and buttonholes. Begin with the shirt completely unbuttoned. The trainer touches the bottom button and says, "JOHN, BUTTON YOUR SHIRT", and immediately assists the resident to align the bottom button with the buttonhole - the resident should then complete action of buttoning. Repeat demonstration with the remainder of the buttons, beginning at the bottom and working up.

Step 5: Terminal behavior: Put the shirt or vest with normal sized buttons and buttonholes on the resident. Begin with the resident's shirt completely unbuttoned. The trainer touches the buttons and says, "JOHN, BUTTON YOUR SHIRT". Give minimal reinforcement and assistance as required.

NOTE: If the resident has difficulty with correct positioning of button and buttonhole; e.g., confusing which button goes with which buttonhole, a shirt marked with colors (bottom button and bottom buttonhole red, next button and buttonhole blue, etc.) may be used. In order to teach correct positioning, the resident may be shown using these color prompts. These prompts should be gradually faded out until the resident reaches criterion with the unmarked shirt.

MODEL LESSON 020
TASK: UNBUTTONING SHIRT

GOAL: Improve dressing skills.

OBJECTIVE: To teach the resident to unbutton his shirt upon request.

MATERIALS: A shirt or vest with large buttons (1½ inch or larger) and buttonholes (½ inch larger than buttons); a shirt or vest with normal size buttons and buttonholes.

SETTING: The resident and trainer sitting, facing each other.

PRE-TEST/ POST-TEST: Put shirt or vest with normal sized buttons and buttonholes on the resident. Begin with the resident's shirt fully buttoned. The trainer touches buttons and says, "JOHN, UNBUTTON YOUR SHIRT". Do not reinforce a correct response and do not correct an incorrect response. Give no assistance.

TEACHING PROCEDURE

STEP 1: Put the shirt or vest with large buttons and buttonholes on the resident in steps 1 through 2. Begin with the bottom button pushed half way out of buttonhole. The trainer says, "JOHN, UNBUTTON YOUR SHIRT", and immediately assists the resident to (a) grasp the left edge of button with his left thumb and forefinger and push that button clear of the buttonhole and simultaneously to (b) grasp the right edge of that buttonhole with his right thumb and forefinger and push the buttonhole away from the button. Repeat demonstration with remainder of buttons, beginning at the bottom and working up. (See notes 1 and 2).

STEP 2: Use large buttons and buttonholes. Begin with the bottom button pushed half way out of the buttonhole, the trainer says, "JOHN, UNBUTTON YOUR SHIRT", and immediately assists the resident to (a) grasp the left edge of the button with his left thumb and forefinger and push that button clear of the buttonhole and simultaneously to (b) grasp the right edge of that buttonhole with his right thumb and forefinger and push the buttonhole away from the buttons, beginning at the bottom and working up. (See notes 1 and 2).

STEP 3: Terminal Behavior- Put the shirt or vest with normal sized buttons and buttonholes on the resident. Begin with the resident's shirt fully buttoned. The trainer touches the buttons and says, "JOHN, UNBUTTON YOUR SHIRT". Give minimal reinforcement and assistance required.

NOTE 1: If the resident has difficulty with this task or with subsequent unbuttoning tasks, the trainer should stop work on the step and initiate practice on the more basic skills needed for unbuttoning. The trainer might have the resident practice making simultaneous actions with his hands like, for example, pulling a token with one hand and simultaneously pushing it with the other hand, back and forth in a narrow slot and a piece of cardboard (a prerequisite needed in step 1). Then, if such practice is not sufficient to alleviate the difficulty in the step, the trainer might have the resident do each step of the lesson using a "button board" that is first placed on a table in front of the resident. (This will enable the resident to work away from his body and to see more easily what he is doing). Give the resident steps 1 through 2 using this frame; then, after the resident has mastered this, go back and re-do those steps using the button board turned upside down and placed flat against the resident's stomach so that the buttons will be on the resident's right side and buttonholes on the resident's left side. (This will enable the resident to work near his body, approximating the terminal behavior). Then, after the resident has mastered this, go back and redo steps 1 through 2 using a shirt or vest on the resident.

NOTE 2: At first, the trainer might require the resident to unbutton only one or two buttons per teaching session. Later, the resident should be required to unbutton half of the buttons on his shirt or vest, and then all the buttons.

MODEL LESSON 021
TASK: SNAPPING SHIRT

GOAL: Improve dressing skills.

OBJECTIVE: To teach the resident to snap shirt or vest upon request.

MATERIALS: A shirt or vest with large plastic "easy to snap" snaps; A shirt or vest with normal size metal snaps.

SETTING: The resident and trainer sitting, facing each other.

PRE-TEST/POST-TEST: Put the shirt or vest with normal size metal snaps on the resident. Begin with the resident's shirt completely unsnapped. The trainer touches the snaps and says, "JOHN, SNAP YOUR SHIRT". Do not reinforce a correct response and do not correct an incorrect response. Give no assistance.

TEACHING PROCEDURE

STEP 1: Put a shirt or vest with large plastic snaps on the resident in steps 1 through 4. Begin with the bottom snap loosened, but not completely snapped, the trainer says, "JOHN, SNAP YOUR SHIRT", and immediately assists the resident to (a) place his forefingers on top of the over-snap and to push down, and simultaneously to (b) place his thumbs under the under-snaps and to push up. Those simultaneous actions will snap the shirt. Repeat demonstration with the remainder of the snaps, beginning at the bottom and working up.

STEP 2: Use "easy to snap" snaps. Begin with the shirt completely unsnapped. The trainer positions bottom snap so that the over-snap is directly on top of the under-snap. The trainer says, "JOHN, SNAP YOUR SHIRT", and immediately assists the resident to complete the action of snapping. Repeat the demonstration with the remainder of the snaps, beginning at the bottom and working up.

STEP 3: Use "easy to snap" snaps. Begin with the shirt completely unsnapped. The trainer aligns the bottom edges of the shirt so that the over-snap is next to the under-snap. The trainer says, "JOHN, SNAP YOUR SHIRT", and immediately assists the resident to place the over-snap directly on top of the under-snap. The resident should then complete the action of snapping. Repeat the demonstration with the complete action of snapping. Repeat the demonstration with the remainder of the snaps, beginning at the bottom and working up.

STEP 4: Use "easy to snap" snaps. Begin with the shirt completely unsnapped. The trainer says, "JOHN, SNAP YOUR SHIRT", and immediately assists the resident to align the bottom edges of the shirt so that the over-snap is next to the under-snap. The resident should then complete the action of snapping. Repeat the demonstration with the remainder of the snaps, beginning at the bottom and working up. (See note 1, 2, and 3.)

STEP 5: Terminal behavior: Put the shirt or vest with normal size metal snaps on the resident. Begin with the resident's shirt completely unsnapped. The trainer touches the snaps and says, "JOHN, SNAP YOUR SHIRT". Give minimal reinforcement and assistance as required.

NOTE 1: If the resident has difficulty with correct positioning of the over-snap and under-snap; e.g., confusing which over-snap goes with which under-snap, a shirt marked with colors (bottom over-snap and bottom under-snap red, next over-snap and under-snap blue, etc.) may be used. In order to teach correct positioning, the resident may be shown how to align the over- snap with the appropriate under-snap using these color prompts. These prompts should be gradually faded out until the resident reaches criterion with the unmarked shirt.

NOTE 2: If the resident has difficulty with this task or with subsequent snapping tasks, the trainer should stop working on this step and initiate practice on the more basic skills needed for pushing plastic pop beads together. Then, if such practice is not sufficient to alleviate the difficulty in this step, the trainer might have the resident to do each step of the lesson plan using a "snap board" that is first placed on a table in front of the resident. Give the resident steps 1 through 4 using this frame; and then, after the resident has mastered this, go back and re-do those steps using the snap board turned upside down and placed flat against the resident's stomach so that the over-snaps will be on the resident's left side and the under-snaps on the resident's right side (this will enable the resident to work near his body, approximating the terminal behavior). Then, after the resident has mastered this, go back and redo steps 1 through 4 using a shirt or vest on the resident.

NOTE 3: At first, the trainer might require the resident to snap only one or two snaps per teaching session. Later, the resident should be required to snap half of the snaps on his shirt or vest, then all of the snaps.

MODEL LESSON 022
TASK: UNSNAPPING SHIRT

GOAL: Improve dressing skills.

OBJECTIVE: To teach the resident to unsnap shirt upon request.

MATERIALS: A shirt or vest with large plastic "easy to snap" snaps; a shirt or vest with normal size metal snaps.

SETTING: The resident and trainer, sitting, facing each other.

PRE-TEST/ POST-TEST: Put shirt or vest with normal size metal snaps on the resident. Begin with the resident's shirt fully snapped. The trainer touches snaps and says, "JOHN, UNSNAP YOUR SHIRT". Do not reinforce a correct response and do not correct an incorrect response. Give no assistance.

TEACHING PROCEDURE

STEP 1: Put the shirt or vest with large plastic snaps on the resident in steps 1 through 2. Begin with the bottom snap loosened, but not completely unsnapped. The trainer says, "JOHN, UNSNAP YOUR SHIRT", and immediately assists the resident to (a) grasp the material at the right edge of the over snap with his left thumb and forefinger and pull it away from the resident's body and simultaneously to (b) grasp the material at the right edge of the under snap with his right thumb and forefinger and hold it down against the resident's stomach. Those simultaneous actions will unsnap the shirt or vest. Repeat the demonstration with the remainder of the snaps, beginning at the bottom and working up.

STEP 2: Use "easy to snap" snaps. Begin with bottom snap completely snapped. The trainer says, "JOHN, UNSNAP YOUR SHIRT", and immediately assists the resident to complete the action of unsnapping. Repeat the demonstration with the remainder of snaps, beginning at the bottom and working up.

STEP 3: Terminal Behavior: Put shirt or vest with normal size metal snaps on the resident. Begin with the resident's shirt fully snapped. The trainer snaps and says, "JOHN, UNSNAP YOUR SHIRT". Give minimal reinforcement and assistance as required.

NOTE 1: If the resident has difficulty with correct positioning of over-snap and under-snap, e.g., confusing which over-snap goes with which under-snap, a shirt marked with colors (bottom over-snap and bottom under snap- red, next over-snap and under-snap blue, etc.) may be used. In order to teach correct positioning, the resident may be shown how to align the over-snap with the appropriate under-snap using these color prompts. These prompts should be gradually faded out until the resident reaches the criterion with the unmarked shirt.

NOTE 2: If the resident has difficulty with this task or with subsequent unsnapping tasks, the resident should stop working on the step and initiate practice on the more basic skills needed for unsnapping. The trainer might have the resident practice pushing plastic pop beads together. Then, if such practice is not sufficient to alleviate the difficulty in the step, the trainer might have the resident do each step of lesson plan using a "snap board" that is first placed on a table in front of the resident. Give the resident steps 1 through 4 using this frame; then, after the resident has mastered this, go back and re-do those steps using the snap board turned upside down and placed flat against the resident's stomach so that the over-snaps will be on the resident's left side and the under-snaps on the resident's right side (this will enable the resident to work near his body, approximating the terminal behavior). Then, after the resident has mastered this, go back and re-do steps 1 through 4 using a shirt or vest on the resident.

NOTE 3: At first, the trainer might require the resident to unsnap only one or two snaps per teaching session. Later, the resident should be required to unsnap half of the snaps on his shirt or vest, and then all of the snaps.

MODEL LESSON 023
TASK: TYING SHOE

GOAL: Improve dressing skills.

OBJECTIVE: To teach the resident to tie his shoe lace upon request.

MATERIALS: The resident's shoe, laced with a long, wide shoe lace. (One end of the shoe lace is white, the other is colored black); the resident's shoe laced with a normal size shoe lace (both laced ends are the same color).

SETTING: The resident and the trainer sitting, facing each other.

PRE-TEST/POST-TEST: Use normal size shoe lace; both laced ends are the same color. Begin with the resident's shoe lace untied. The trainer touches the laced ends and says, "JOHN, TIE YOUR SHOE". Do not reinforce a correct a correct response and do not correct an incorrect response. Give no assistance.

TEACHING PROCEDURE

STEP 1: Use oversize shoe lace; each laced and is a different color, in steps 1 through 5. Begin with laced and tied and bowed, very loosely. The trainer says, "JOHN, TIE YOUR SHOE LACE", and immediately assists the resident to (a) grasp the right loop of the shoe lace with his right thumb and forefinger and the left loop with his left thumb and forefinger and, (b) to pull the loop out and away from each other so that the bow is tightened.

STEP 2: Use oversize shoe lace. Begin with the laced ends tied and one laced loop just pushed through the opening of the loop to form a knot. The trainer says, "JOHN, TIE YOUR SHOE LACE", and immediately assists the resident to grasp both loops with respective thumbs and forefingers and to pull loops out so the bow is tightened.

STEP 3: Use oversized shoe lace. Begin with laced ends tied, but not bowed. The trainer forms a loop with each laced end. The trainer forms a loop with each laced end. The trainer says, "JOHN, TIE YOUR SHOE LACE", and immediately assists the resident to cross loops and push one loop behind and through the opening to form a knot. The resident should then complete action to tighten the bow.

STEP 4: Use oversized shoe lace. Begin with the lace tied, but not bowed. The trainer says, "JOHN, TIE YOUR SHOE LACE", and immediately assists the resident to form a loop with each lace end. The resident should then complete action to form and tighten the bow.

STEP 5: Use over sized shoe lace. Begin with the laces untied. The trainer says, "JOHN, TIE YOUR SHOE LACE", and immediately assists the resident to cross the lace ends, tie them, and pull them out with respective thumbs and forefingers so that the tie is tightened. The resident should then complete action to form and to tighten the bow.

STEP 6: Terminal Behavior - Use normal size shoe lace; both laced ends are the same color. Begin with the resident's shoe lace untied. The trainer touches laced ends and says, "JOHN, TIE YOUR SHOE LACE" (see note 1).

Give minimal reinforcement and assistance as required.

NOTE 1: If the resident has difficulty at this step, the trainer should return to step 5 and gradually fade out the first color prompt (making the laced ends more and more similar in color) and then the size also (making the lace closer and closer to normal size).

NOTE 2: The trainer may wish to teach to tie shoe using the alternative method of making one loop, passing the other laced end around that loop and pushing it through the hole, thus formed so that another loop is formed and the bow can be tightened. This sequence of tasks should be broken down into several sub-tasks and presented to the resident as a backward chain, as is done in this lesson plan.

MODEL LESSON 024
TASK: UNTYING SHOE.

GOAL: Improve dressing skills.

OBJECTIVE: To teach the resident to untie his shoe lace upon request.

MATERIALS: A shoe, laced with a long, wide shoe lace (one end of the lace is white, the other a normal size lace (both laced ends are the same color).

SETTING: The resident and trainer sitting, facing each other.

PRE-TEST/POST-TEST: Use normal size shoe lace: both laced ends are the same color. Begin with the resident's shoe lace tied and bowed. The trainer touches laced ends and says, "JOHN, UNTIE YOUR SHOE". Do not reinforce a correct response and do not correct an incorrect response. Give no assistance.

TEACHING PROCEDURE

STEP 1: Use over-sized shoe lace; each laced and is a different color, in steps 1 through 3. Begin with laced ends tied, but not bowed. The trainer says, "JOHN, UNTIE YOUR SHOE LACE", and immediately assists the resident to place his right index finger under the tied laced ends and pull up until the ends are pulled apart.

STEP 2: Use over-sized shoe lace. Begin with the laced ends tied very loosely. The trainer says, "JOHN, UNTIE YOUR SHOE LACE", and immediately assists the resident to (a) grasp right hand of lace with right thumb and forefinger and left hand with left thumb and forefinger and (b) to pull lace ends out and away from each other so the bow is untied. The resident should then complete action to untie the lace.

STEP 3: Use oversize shoe lace. Begin with laced ends tied and bowed tightly. The trainer says, "JOHN, UNTIE YOUR SHOE LACE", and immediately assists the resident to complete action to untie the lace.

STEP 4: Terminal Behavior - Use normal size shoe lace; both laced ends are the same color. Begin with the resident's shoe laces tied and bowed. The trainer touches the laced ends and says, "JOHN, UNTIE YOUR SHOE LACE". (See Note 1).

NOTE 1. If the resident has difficulty at this step, the trainer should return to step 3 and then gradually fade out the first color prompt (making the laced ends more and more similar in color) and then the size cue (making the lace closer and closer to the normal size).

MODEL LESSON 025
TASK: BRA – HOOKING

GOAL: Improve dressing skills.

OBJECTIVE: To teach the resident to hook bra upon request. (See Note 1).

MATERIALS: The resident's normal sized bra.

SETTING: The resident sits or stands near the trainer.

PRE-TEST/POST-TEST: Use normal size bra. Begin with the bra off the resident. The trainer puts the ringed end of the bra in the resident's right hand which is resting on her stomach. The trainer then wraps hooked end around the resident, and places it in the resident's hand which is also resting on her stomach (see notes 1 and 2). This procedure should be carried out for all steps (steps 1 through 5). The trainer touches the hooks and says, "JANE, HOOK YOUR BRA". Do not reinforce a correct response and do not correct response. Give no assistance.

TEACHING PROCEDURE

STEP 1: Use resident's normal size bra throughout. Begin with the bottom edges of the bra with the bottom hook loosened but not completely hooked. The trainer says, "JANE, HOOK YOUR BRA", and immediately assists the resident to (a) place her thumb and forefinger around the hooked end and push to the left and simultaneously, (b) to place her thumb and forefinger around the ringed end and push to the right. These simultaneous actions will hook the bra ends. Repeat demonstration with the remainder of the hooks, beginning at the bottom and working up.

STEP 2: Begin with the bra ends completely unhooked. The trainer positions the ringed end so that the bottom hooked end is directed on top of the ringed end. The trainer says, "JANE, HOOK YOUR BRA", and immediately assists the resident to complete the action of hooking. Repeat the demonstration with the remainder of the hooks, beginning at the bottom and working up.

STEP 3: Begin with the bra ends completely unhooked. The trainer aligns the bottom edges of the bra ends so that the hooked end is next to the ringed end. The trainer says, "JANE, HOOK YOUR BRA", and immediately assists the resident to place the bottom hooked end directly over and slightly to the right of the ringed end. The resident should then complete the action of hooking the bra. Repeat the demonstration with the remainder of the hooks, beginning at the bottom and working up.

STEP 4: Demonstration - Begin with the bra ends completely unhooked. The trainer says, "JANE, HOOK YOUR BRA", and immediately assists the resident to align the bottom of the bra ends so that the hooked end is next to the ringed end. The resident should then complete the action of hooking the bra. Repeat the demonstration with the remainder of the hooks, beginning at the bottom and working up.

STEP 5: Terminal Behavior - Use normal sized bra (see Note 3). Begin with the bra ends completely unhooked. The trainer touches the hooks and says, "JANE, HOOK YOUR BRA". Give minimal reinforcement and assistance as required.

NOTE 1: If the resident has difficulty with the correct positioning of the hooked end and ringed end confusing which hooked end goes with which ringed end, a bra marked with colors (bottom hooked end and bottom ringed end red, next hooked end and ringed blue, etc.) may be used. In order to teach correct positioning, the resident may be shown how to align the hooked end with the appropriate ringed end using these color prompts. Those prompts should be gradually faded out until the resident reaches the criterion with the unmarked bra.

NOTE 2: If the resident has difficulty in learning the bra hooking, dressing procedure, the trainer might have the resident do each step of the lesson plan using a "snap board" that is first placed on a table on front of the resident, positioned in the same manner as if she were putting on her own bra. That is, the hooked ends are on the left and the ringed ends are on the right side of the board. (This will enable the resident to work away from her body to see more easily what she is doing). The snap-board would be made by cutting off the ends of a bra and attaching them to a wooden frame so that all the sides are secure except the two one (1) inch edges upon which two rows of ringed ends and one column of hooked ends are mounted.

NOTE 3: After the resident has passed step 6 (terminal behavior and post-test) of the bra hooking, dressing procedure, the resident should then be put into the regular bra-dressing procedure program.

MODEL LESSON 026
TASK: BRA UNHOOKING.

GOAL: Improve dressing skills.

OBJECTIVE: To teach the resident to unhook bra upon request.

MATERIALS: The resident's normal size bra; with hook and ring ends.

SETTING: The resident sits or stands, the trainer stands near the resident.

PRE-TEST/ POST-TEST: Use normal size bra. Begin with bra ends completely hooked and around the resident's waist. The trainer hooks and says, "JANE, UNHOOK YOUR BRA". Do not reinforce a correct response and do not correct an incorrect response. Give no assistance.

TEACHING PROCEDURE

STEP 1: Demonstration - Use normal size bra. Begin with the top edges of the bra with the top hook loosened but not completely unhooked (if possible). The trainer says, "JANE, UNHOOK YOUR BRA", and immediately assists the resident to (a) place her thumb and forefinger around the hooked end and push to the right and simultaneously, (b) to place her thumb and forefinger around the ringed end and push to the left. These simultaneous actions will unhook the bra ends. Repeat the demonstration with the remainder of the hooks, beginning at the top and working down.

STEP 2: Terminal Behavior - Begin with the bra with ends completely hooked. The trainer touches the hooks and says, "JANE, UNHOOK YOUR BRA". Give minimal reinforcement and assistance as required.

CHAPTER FIVE

MODEL PLANS

TABLE OF CONTENTS

DINING BEHAVIOR CHECKLIST

RESIDENT _____NO._____DATE_____

EVALUATOR_____ROOM _____

RATING:

1. Never been observed to perform the skill by him or herself, even though he or she has had the opportunity.

2. Does task sometimes by him or herself, but not adequately (sloppy, because he or she does not know how - this means that you have never seen him or her do it correctly at least once, but he or she tries).

3. Performs the task adequately with verbal assistance (if someone tells him or her to do it or how to do it).

4. Does it sometimes by him or herself but not adequately (sloppy), but he or she does know how - this means that you have seen him or her do it correctly at least once.

5. Performs the task adequately and consistently (most of the time) without verbal or physical assistance.

N.O. - No opportunity to perform the task.

P.D. - Does not do because physically disabled.

BASELINE + = does it alone.

O = does not do it.

- = needs help.

Behavior / Step or task	Rating	Date	Date	Date	Date	Date	Date	Date
1. Enters dining room	——	——	——	——	——	——	——	——
2. Goes through line	——	——	——	——	——	——	——	——
3. Picks up tray	——	——	——	——	——	——	——	——
4. Picks up utensil	——	——	——	——	——	——	——	——
5. Selects food items	——	——	——	——	——	——	——	——
6. Selects glass and drink	——	——	——	——	——	——	——	——
7. Carries tray	——	——	——	——	——	——	——	——
8. Selects table	——	——	——	——	——	——	——	——
9. Stands behind chair	——	——	——	——	——	——	——	——
10. Places tray on table	——	——	——	——	——	——	——	——
11. Pulls chair out from table	——	——	——	——	——	——	——	——
12. Sits down	——	——	——	——	——	——	——	——

13. Pulls
him or
herself to
table   —— —— —— —— —— —— —— ——

14. Uses
spoon to
eat   —— —— —— —— —— —— —— ——

15. Uses
fork to eat —— —— —— —— —— —— —— ——

16. Uses
knife to cut —— —— —— —— —— —— —— ——

17. Drinks
from glass   —— —— —— —— —— —— —— ——

18. Cleans
table area   —— —— —— —— —— —— —— ——

19. Pushes
chair back
from table   —— —— —— —— —— —— —— ——

20. Stands
up from
table   —— —— —— —— —— —— —— ——

21. Puts
chair back
under table —— —— —— —— —— —— —— ——

22. Picks
up tray   —— —— —— —— —— —— —— ——

23. Takes
tray to
dishwasher   —— —— —— —— —— —— —— ——
station

24. Empties tray at station _____ _____ _____ _____ _____ _____ _____ _____

25. Empties tray at station _____ _____ _____ _____ _____ _____ _____ _____

26. Leaves dining room _____ _____ _____ _____ _____ _____ _____ _____

DINING PROGRAM

PROBLEM BEHAVIOR BASELINE

RESIDENT _____NO. _____ DATE_____

EVALUATOR _____ROOM _____

BEHAVIOR/STEP-TASK	Date	Date	Date	Date	Date	Date	Date
1. Eats too slowly	____	____	____	____	____	____	____
2. Eats too quickly	____	____	____	____	____	____	____
3. Refuses to eat	____	____	____	____	____	____	____
4. Fills mouth too full	____	____	____	____	____	____	____
5. Taps spoon on dish/table	____	____	____	____	____	____	____
6. Eats with fingers	____	____	____	____	____	____	____
7. Drinks from glass with one hand, eats food with other hand.	____	____	____	____	____	____	____
8. Uses both hands to eat or drink	____	____	____	____	____	____	____
9. Spills food/drink	____	____	____	____	____	____	____
10. Sits improperly	____	____	____	____	____	____	____
11. Chews food improperly	____	____	____	____	____	____	____
12. Swallows food whole	____	____	____	____	____	____	____

13. Throws food utensils   —— —— —— —— —— —— ——

14. Eats food from table/floor   —— —— —— —— —— —— ——

15. Spits food out of mouth   —— —— —— —— —— —— ——

16. Steals food   —— —— —— —— —— —— ——

17. Burps at table   —— —— —— —— —— —— ——

18. Brings objects to table   —— —— —— —— —— —— ——

19. Drools   —— —— —— —— —— —— ——

20. Licks food from plate/table   —— —— —— —— —— —— ——

21. Plays in food   —— —— —— —— —— —— ——

22. Rubs food on body   —— —— —— —— —— —— ——

LIST ANY ADAPTIVE FEEDING DEVICES REQUIRED.

1._____

2._____

3._____

4._____

5._____

6._____

7._____

8._____

DINING PROGRAM

Dining, with the exception of those behaviors for which specific training routines have been developed (e.g., spoon feeding), the behaviors in the sequence will be taught by using general shaping, graduated guidance, modeling and reinforcement procedures. The trainer should select the procedures best suited to the performance level of the resident. In some instances manual guidance may be the most appropriate. In other instances where the resident has demonstrated that they can imitate a modeled behavior, modeling and manual guidance may be more effective.

In training those behaviors for which specific procedures have not been outlined, the dining program training sheet will be used. The trainer will begin with the first step in the sequence by targeting that step for shaping and reinforcement. Reinforcement in this case will be one small bite of some edible that the resident has demonstrated that he or she likes. If the resident responds in the required manner or has been given a demonstrated trial on the targeted behavior, he or she will get the reinforcement. Due to the nature of the training session (meal time) no more than one (1) trial will be reinforced per session to avoid interfering with the resident's appetite. The trainer should, however, dispense emphatic social praise for correct or prompted performance in the manner described in the general procedures section. Give social praise in the following manner, "Good job, John or Jane", "You're eating with a fork, etc."

On the data sheet, check the step that is currently targeted (being worked on). If the resident does it alone, enter a plus (+). If he or she does it if you assist or manually guide him or her, enter a minus (-). If he or she will not do it at all (resists) enter a zero (0). As soon as the resident performs the task correctly three (3) times in a row, put a plus (+) in the first column (overriding the check mark) and target the next behavior. As soon as the resident begins to respond correctly on the next step require him or her to correctly complete on the step and only that he or she has complete sequences should be chained together in this manner. More potent reinforcement may be needed at this point, however, so consult with the professional personnel for further instruction.

Data on these behaviors for which specific procedures are available will be recorded on the standard training program stage analysis data sheet.

DINING PROGRAM TRAINING SHEET

**Check if behavior
is to be targeted:
Plus (+) if completed,
Minus (-) if not completed.**

DAILY DATE

Date Date   Date Date Date

BEHAVIOR

1. _____ Enters dining room   ___ ___ ___ ___ ___
2. _____ Goes through line   ___ ___ ___ ___ ___
3. _____ Picks up tray   ___ ___ ___ ___ ___
4. _____ Picks up utensils   ___ ___ ___ ___ ___
5. _____ Selects food items   ___ ___ ___ ___ ___
6. _____ Gets glass & drink   ___ ___ ___ ___ ___
7. _____ Carries tray   ___ ___ ___ ___ ___
8. _____ Selects table   ___ ___ ___ ___ ___
9. _____ Stands behind chair   ___ ___ ___ ___ ___
10. _____ Sets tray down   ___ ___ ___ ___ ___
11. _____ Pulls chair out   ___ ___ ___ ___ ___
12. _____ Sits down   ___ ___ ___ ___ ___
13. _____ Pulls self to table   ___ ___ ___ ___ ___
14. _____ Cleans table area   ___ ___ ___ ___ ___
15. _____ Pushes chair back   ___ ___ ___ ___ ___
16. _____ Stands up from table   ___ ___ ___ ___ ___
17. _____ Pushes chair under table___ ___ ___ ___ ___
18. _____ Picks up tray   ___ ___ ___ ___ ___
19. _____ Takes tray to station   ___ ___ ___ ___ ___
20. _____ Empties tray at station   ___ ___ ___ ___ ___
21. _____ Leaves dining area   ___ ___ ___ ___ ___

MODEL LESSON 101
TASK: UTENSIL TRAINING - SPOON FEEDING

GOAL: Improve dining skills.

OBJECTIVE: To teach the resident to use spoon properly and neatly without assistance.

MATERIALS: A plate with spoon, foods which the resident will readily eat. Examples include cut-up pieces of fruit, pieces of meat, soup, soft foods, i.e., noodles, and spoon vegetables.

SETTING: Meal time. The resident is before him or her. The trainer stands behind the resident.

TEACHING PROCEDURE

The following teaching/training procedures will apply for steps 1 through 9. The steps are defined below in the naturally occurring order (forward chaining).

1. Picking up spoon and forming hand correctly around it.

2. Holding the spoon in his or her hand.

3. Dipping the spoon in the food.

4. Scooping the food onto the spoon.

5. Lift the filled spoon toward the mouth.

6. Move the filled spoon to position at mouth, approximately two (2) inches from his or her mouth.

7. Open mouth by placing left hand on the resident's chin and gently open his or her mouth.

8. Put filled spoon in the resident's mouth.

9. Guiding the resident's hand upward and outward resulting in the food being removed from the spoon by the resident's upper teeth or lip.

Beginning with Step 1, the trainer will demonstrate procedure by physically prompting the resident to complete the entire nine (9) step sequence. Incorporate graduated guidance procedures even at this early stage, i.e., use only enough physical prompting to get the resident to perform the task. Each Training Step is set up on the basis of complete withdrawal of assistance at a specified point in the sequence. Thus, after the resident has gone through the entire nine (9) step sequence, on each trial, the trainer then assists the resident to complete every step up to the step outlined as the stage for training. Immediately prior to that step, the trainer will with-draw assistance so that the resident must complete that behavior (as well as previously learned behaviors) to obtain reinforcement and receive a plus (+) mark on the data sheet for the task request. If the resident performs incorrectly or not at all then the trainer assists the resident to complete the stage and makes the appropriate entry on the data sheet.

STEPS FOR TRAINING

STEP 1: The trainer withdraws assistance after step eight (8) - putting spoon in mouth of resident who must empty contents into mouth on his or her own.

STEP 2: The trainer withdraws assistance after step seven (7) - opening mouth. The resident must put spoon in mouth and empty contents.

STEP 3: The trainer withdraws assistance after step six (6) - positioning spoon at mouth.

STEP 4: The trainer withdraws assistance after step five (5) - lifting spoon toward mouth.

STEP 5: The trainer withdraws assistance after step four (4) - scooping food onto spoon.

STEP 6: The trainer withdraws assistance after step three (3) - dipping spoon in food.

STEP 7: The trainer withdraws assistance after step two (2) - holding spoon in hand.

STEP 8: The trainer withdraws assistance after step one (1) - picking up spoon and forming hand correctly around it.

STEP 9: Terminal Behavior. The resident must correctly perform the complete nine (9) step sequence.

MODEL PLAN 102
TASK: UTENSIL TRAINING – FORK FEEDING

GOAL: Improve dining skills.

OBJECTIVE: To teach the resident to use a fork properly, and neatly, without assistance.

MATERIALS: A plate with fork foods which the resident will readily eat. Examples include cut-up pieces of fruit, pieces of meat, soft food, i.e., noodles and "fork" vegetables.

SETTING: Mealtime. The resident is seated and the tray of only fork foods is before him or her.

TEACHING PROCEDURE

The following Teaching Procedures will apply for steps one (1) through eight (8). The steps are defined below in the naturally occurring order (forward chaining).

1. Picking up the fork and forming hand correctly around it.

2. Holding fork in hand.

3. Spearing/scooping the food with the fork.

4. Lifting the fork with food toward the mouth.

5. Moving the fork with food to position at mouth, within two inches of mouth.

6. Opening mouth by placing left hand on resident's chin and gently opening mouth.

7. Putting fork with food in mouth.

8. Guiding resident's hand upward and outward resulting in the food being removed from the fork by resident's upper teeth or lip.

Beginning with step 1, the trainer will demonstrate by physically assisting the resident to complete the entire eight (8) step sequence. Incorporate graduated guidance procedures even at this early stage, i.e., use only enough physical prompts to get the resident to perform the task. Each Training Stage is set up on the basis of complete withdrawal of assistance of a specified point in the sequence. Thus, after the resident has gone through the entire 8 step sequence, on each trial, the trainer then assists the resident to complete every step up to the step outlined as the step for training. Immediately prior to that step, the trainer will withdraw assistance so that the resident must complete that behavior (as well as previously learned behaviors) to obtain reinforcement and receive a plus (+) on the data sheet for task request. If the resident responds incorrectly or not at all, then the trainer assists the resident to complete the step and makes the appropriate entry on the data sheet.

STEPS FOR TRAINING

STEP 1: The trainer withdraws assistance after step 7 - putting fork with food in mouth.

STEP 2: The trainer withdraws assistance after step 6 - moving the fork to position at mouth. The resident must complete steps 7 and 8.

STEP 3: The trainer withdraws assistance after step 5 - moving fork with food to position at mouth. The resident must complete step 6 through 8.

STEP 4: The trainer withdraws assistance after step 4 - lifting fork toward the mouth. The resident must complete steps 5 through 8.

STEP 5: The trainer withdraws assistance after step 3 - spearing/scooping food onto fork. The resident must complete steps 4 through 8.

STEP 6: The trainer withdraws assistance after step 2 - holding fork in hand. The resident must complete steps 3 through 8.

STEP 7: The trainer withdraws assistance after step 1 - picking up fork and forming hand correctly around it. The resident must complete steps 2 through 8.

STEP 8: Terminal Behavior. The resident must correctly perform entire 8 step sequence beginning with picking up fork and forming hand correctly around it.

MODEL LESSON 103
TASK: UTENSIL TRAINING – GLASS DRINKING

GOAL: Improve dining skills.

OBJECTIVE: To teach the resident to use a glass properly, and neatly, with one hand, (if physically able) without assistance.

MATERIALS: A glass filled with liquid edibles.

SETTING: Mealtime. The resident is seated at the table and a glass of liquid drink is presented with his or her meal. The trainer stands behind him or her.

TEACHING PROCEDURE

The following Teaching Procedure will apply for steps 1 through 7. The steps are defined below in the naturally occurring order (forward chaining).

1. Gripping glass securely with one hand.

2. Lifting the glass (filled) toward mouth.

3. Moving the filled glass to position at mouth, approximately one inch from mouth.

4. Opening mouth. The trainer may have to assist by placing his or her left hand on the resident's chin and gently opening mouth.

5. Putting rim of glass over bottom lip.

6. Lifting lower part of the glass so that the liquid flows into mouth at a rate at which there is no spilling.

7. Putting glass down.

Beginning with step 1, the trainer will demonstrate by physically assisting the resident to complete the entire seven step sequence. Incorporate graduated guidance procedures even at this early stage, i.e., use only enough physical prompts to get the resident to do the task. Each training step is set up on the basis of complete withdrawal of assistance at a specified point in the sequence. Thus, after the resident has gone through the entire seven step sequence, on each trial, the trainer then assists the resident to complete every step up to the step outlined as the step for training. Immediately prior to that step, the trainer will withdraw assistance so that the resident must complete that behavior (as well as previously learned behaviors) to obtain reinforcement and receive a plus (+) mark on the data sheet for task request. If the resident performs incorrectly or not at all, then the trainer assists the resident to complete the step and makes the appropriate entry, a minus (-), on data sheet.

STEPS FOR TRAINING

STEP 1: The trainer withdraws assistance after step 6 - lifting the lower part of the glass so that the liquid flows into mouth at a rate at which there is no spillage. The resident must set glass down independently.

STEP 2: The trainer withdraws assistance after step 5 putting the rim of drinking glass over bottom lip. The resident must lift the lower part of the glass so that the liquid flows into mouth at a rate at which there is no spillage, and then set the glass down.

STEP 3: The trainer withdraws assistance after step 4 opening mouth.

STEP 4: The trainer withdraws assistance after step 3 moving the filled glass to position at mouth, approximately one inch from mouth.

STEP 5: The trainer withdraws assistance after step 2 lifting the glass (filled) towards mouth.

STEP 6: The trainer withdraws assistance after step 1 gripping glass securely with one hand.

STEP 7: Terminal Behavior. The resident must correctly perform the complete seven step sequence.

MODEL LESSON 104
TASK: UTENSIL TRAINING – KNIFE FEEDING <u>(SPREADING)</u>

GOAL: Improve dining skills.

OBJECTIVE: To teach the resident to use a knife to spread soft foods on bread, neatly, without assistance.

MATERIALS: A knife with either slices of bread, rolls, biscuits or buns included with regular meal. Also, near hand is either margarine, jelly, butter, cheese spread, or peanut butter on the side of plate.

SETTING: Mealtime. The resident is seated and his meal is before him or her. The trainer stands behind resident.

TEACHING PROCEDURE

The following Teaching Procedure will apply for steps 1 through 9. These steps are defined below in the naturally occurring order (forward chaining).

1. Pick up sliced bread with preferred hand and secure it in the other hand, such that it is in a position for spreading.

2. With preferred hand, secure knife appropriately.

3. Dip knife in soft spread.

4. Cover knife blade with the spread and lift it from spread.

5. Take knife with spread over toward bread.

6. Lay knife with spread on area of bread further from the knife hand.

7. Spread in one smooth stroke from outside area of bread to inside area.

8. Lay knife down.

9. "Change hands", so that the preferred hand is holding the bread securely.

Beginning with step 1, the trainer will demonstrate by physically assisting the resident to complete the entire nine step sequence. Incorporate graduated guidance procedures even at this early stage, i.e., use only enough physical prompts to get the resident to perform the task. Each training step is set up on the basis complete withdrawal of assistance at a specified point in the sequence. Thus, after the resident has gone through the entire nine step sequence, on each trial, the trainer then assists the resident to complete every step up to the step outlined as the stage for training.

Immediately prior to that step, the trainer will withdraw assistance so that the resident must complete that behavior (as well as previously learned behaviors) to obtain reinforcement and receive a plus (+ mark) on the data sheet for task request. If the resident performs incorrectly or not at all, then the trainer assists the resident to complete the step and make the appropriate entry, a minus (-), on data sheet.

STEPS FOR TRAINING

STEP 1: The trainer withdraws assistance after step 8 and sets knife down. The resident must "change hands" so that the preferred hand is holding the bread securely.

STEP 2: The trainer withdraws assistance after step 7 to spread in one smooth stroke from outside area of bread to inside area. The resident must set knife down, and "change hands", so that preferred hand is holding the bread securely.

STEP 3: The trainer withdraws assistance after step 6 to lay knife with spread on area of bread further from the knife hand.

STEP 4: The trainer withdraws assistance after step 5 to take knife with spread over toward bread.

Step 5: The trainer withdraws assistance after step 4 to cover knife blade with the spread and lift it from spread.

STEP 6: The trainer withdraws assistance after step 3 to dip knife in soft spread.

STEP 7: The trainer withdraws assistance after step 2 (with preferred hand). Secure knife appropriately.

STEP 8: The trainer withdraws assistance after step 1 to pick up sliced bread with preferred hand and secure it in the other hand, so that it is in a position for spreading.

STEP 9: Terminal Behavior. The resident must correctly perform the complete nine (9) steps sequence.

MODEL LESSON 105:
TASK: UTENSIL TRAINING - KNIFE FEEDING (CUTTING)

GOAL: Improve dining skills.

OBJECTIVE: To teach the resident to use a knife to cut tender meats and other foods, neatly and without assistance.

MATERIALS: A fork, knife, and a plate with tender meats included with regular meal.

SETTING: Mealtime. The resident is seated at table with meal before him or her. The trainer stands behind the resident.

TEACHING PROCEDURES

The following teaching procedures will apply for steps 1 through 4. The steps are defined below in the naturally occurring order (forward chaining).

1. Pick up and hold fork correctly for cutting.

2. Put fork in meat to secure it to plate.

3. Use knife to separate meat into small and smaller pieces until they are bite size.

4. Lift the fork from the meat, and place both the fork and knife down on table.

Beginning with step 1, the trainer will demonstrate by physically assisting the resident to complete the entire four step sequence. Incorporate graduated guidance procedures even at this early stage, i.e., use only enough physical prompts to get the resident to perform the task. Each training step is set up on the basis of complete withdrawal of assistance of a specified point in the sequence. Thus, after the resident has gone through the entire four step sequence, on each trial, the trainer then assists the resident to complete every step up to the step outlined as the stage for training.

Immediately prior to that step, the trainer will withdraw assistance so that the resident must complete that behavior (as well as previously learned behaviors), to obtain reinforcement and receive a plus (+) mark on the data sheet for task request. If the resident performs incorrectly or not at all, then the trainer assists the resident to complete the step and make the appropriate entry, a minus (-), on the data sheet.

STEPS FOR TRAINING

STEP 1: The trainer withdraws assistance after step 3 using the knife to separate the meat into small and smaller pieces until they are bite size. The resident must lift the fork from the meat, and set both the knife and fork down on table.

STEP 2: The trainer withdraws assistance after step 2 to put the fork in the meat to secure it to the plate. The resident must use the knife to separate the meat into small and smaller pieces until they are bite-size. The resident must lift the fork from the meat and set both the knife and fork down on table.

STEP 3: The trainer withdraws assistance after step 1 to pick up and hold knife correctly for cutting.

STEP 4: Terminal Behavior. The resident must correctly perform the complete four step sequence independently.

PROCEDURES FOR PROBLEM BEHAVIORS

1. Behavior - eats too slowly.

Corrective measure: (1) Timer is set for 15 minutes for the main meal and 5 minutes for dessert period. The periods may be longer at first, gradually reducing to shorter periods of time. The resident can learn approximate time allotment for eating by this procedure. (2) The food is removed when the bell ends the eating period. No dessert is given unless a specified portion main meal is completed, and (3) positively reinforce the resident i.e. stroke, pat, rub or say, "That's Good", "You did well", when meal is completed during the time allowed. Reinforce him or her during dessert period.

2. Behavior - eats too quickly.

Corrective measure: (1) If the resident begins to gulp his or her food down, the tray is taken away from the resident for five (5) minutes, (2) when the tray is returned, the resident is told to "eat slowly". (3) If the resident continues to eat at a rate of more than 5 bites per 30 seconds, the tray is again taken away from him or her. This is done as often as necessary, but not to exceed the length of meal time, and (4) the resident is given verbal praise for eating slowly.

3. Behavior - refuses to eat. (a) All food items. Corrective measure:

(1) Decide what reinforcers are appropriate for the resident, (2) offer reinforcement in return for the resident taking one bite of the food of his or her choice, (3) offer reinforcement in return for the resident taking three bites of the food of his or her choice, and, (4) fade out reinforcement.

4. Behavior - refuses to eat. (b) Has low preference for food items. Corrective measure:

(1) Decide the highest preference for food on the plate, i.e., simply watch the resident's selection of first bite, (2) show the resident a teaspoon of high preference food. When he or she eats a bite of undesired food, then the resident is given a spoonful of desired food, and, (3) at first, the resident gets one

bite of desired food for each bite of undesired food. Gradually this (schedule) is altered until the resident can eat more bites of undesired food in exchange for one bite of desired food.

5. Behavior - fills mouth too full. Corrective measure:

Replace hand used for eating in his or her lap after each bite.

6. Behavior - taps spoon, knife or fork on the dish, plate or table. Corrective measure:

Replace eating hand in his or lap after each bite.

7. Behavior - pushes food items onto fork or spoon with his or her fingers (touches food). Corrective method:

Replace preferred hand in his or her lap following each bite.

8. Behavior - drinks liquid from glass with one hand while stuffing food items in his or her mouth with the other hand. Corrective measure:

Place non-preferred hand in his or her lap and replace individual's preference hand in lap following each bite.

9. Behavior - use both hands to eat or drink simultaneously. Corrective measure:

Place non-preferred hand in lap and replace preference hand in lap of resident following each bite.

10. Behavior - spills food off utensil. Corrective measure:

(1) Stop the resident from filling utensil (spoon or fork) too full. (2) Go through motor movement with the resident and then fade assistance, and (3) reinforce appropriate eating and drinking behavior.

11. Behavior - drops food off utensil (unless physically disabled). Corrective measure:

(1) The food is picked up by the resident and put in a pile beside the resident's plate (the resident uses his or her spoon to do this). (2) The resident is then able to return to the plate for food, repeating the process of picking up the food if it is dropped. (3) The resident is not allowed to eat spilled food, and, (4) The resident is praised for taking bites of food without spilling it.

12. Behavior - Sits improperly at table. Corrective measure:

(1) The resident is told to "sit straight" or told to "put feet on the floor", whichever is applicable. (2) The trainer holds the resident's shoulder back and says "hold your head up". Whenever the head is up, the resident is allowed to have a bite of food. The resident is given verbal praise when head is held up. When the head is down the resident is not allowed a bite of food nor is given praise.

13. Behavior - Chews food improperly or swallows it whole. Corrective measure:

(1) Demonstrate - the trainer exhibits or mimics chewing food with his teeth, and says "chew your food". The trainer may place his or her fingers under the resident's chin and rotates jaw, and, (2) practice by chewing gum if the resident doesn't swallow it.

14. Behavior - Throws food or equipment. Corrective measure:

(1) Remove resident's plate immediately. (2) Push resident away from the table, and, (3) reinforce by giving verbal and physical praise for appropriate behavior.

15. Behavior - Eats food off table or floor. Corrective measure:

(1) Push resident away from the table, (2) the trainer then says, "No", and (3) reinforce resident with verbal and physical praise for appropriate behavior.

16. Behavior - Spits food out of mouth or drools while eating. Corrective measure:

(1) Remove or withdraw food from resident's mouth, (2) the trainer may ask, "Do you like your food?" The resident may dislike the food which may cause him or her to spit food out. (3) The trainer will reinforce with verbal and physical praise for appropriate chewing.

17. Behavior - Fails to use napkin to clean mouth and hands. Corrective measure:

(1) The resident is told to "wipe your face and hands", is given a napkin and, (2) the resident is reinforced with verbal and physical praise for voluntary use of the napkin.

18. Behavior - Steals someone else's food. Corrective measure:

(1) The resident's hand is grasped at the wrist during the act, and the food is emptied back into the source from which it came; and at the same time the trainer says, "No!" Maybe the trainer is standing too far away from the resident to grasp his or her hand at the time. In this case, the trainer says "No!", and moves closer to correct the behavior. (2) The resident is told by the trainer to take his or her tray and redirect to another table to complete meal.

19. Behavior - Resident burps at the table. Corrective measure:

(1) The trainer models phrase for the resident and says, "Excuse me, please", and (2) reinforce resident with verbal and physical praise for his or her approximations to phrase.

20. Behavior - Brings non-dining objects to table. Corrective measure:

(1) The resident is allowed to bring an object near his or her table, but not at the table. The resident is rewarded with something he or she likes instead, (2) the resident is allowed to bring object within his or her sight. The resident is rewarded with verbal and physical praise for complying, (3) the resident is allowed to bring object to the dining room, but out of his or her sight. He or she is rewarded with verbal and physical praise for complying, and (4) the resident is not allowed to bring object to dining room. He or she is rewarded with verbal and physical praise when complying with rewards being gradually faded out.

21. Behavior - Licks food from other objects other than lips.
Corrective measure:

(1) The resident is told to "stop". The resident is then handed a napkin and told to wipe his mouth.

22. Behavior - Rubs spilled liquid or food on his or her face, arms or hands. Corrective measure:

(1) The resident is told to "stop", then the resident is handed a napkin and told to wipe his or her skin clean. (2) The resident is then excused from the table and is sent to the bathroom where he or she washes his or her hands,

and, (3) he or she is then returned to the dining area and allowed to continue eating if there is still food on his or her plate. If not, he or she is told to put up his or her tray.

23. Behavior - Playing with food. Corrective measure:

(1) The resident's tray (meal) is removed for five (5) minutes (the resident is obviously not through eating). The resident's tray (meal) is removed for the day if the resident is through eating. (2) The resident is reinforced with verbal and physical praise for appropriate meal time behavior.

BEHAVIORAL DEFINITIONS OF FEEDING RESPONSES

1. Spoon Response: Moving appropriate food from the container (i.e., pudding, soup) with the spoon held in one hand, by the handle, right side up and without spilling, except back into the container from which it was taken.

2. Glass Response: Moving glass with one hand and without spilling.

3. Food Response: Moving appropriate food from the container (i.e., meat, beans) with the fork held in one hand by the handle, right side up and without spilling, except back into the container from which the food was taken.

4. Hand Response: Moving appropriate food from the container (i.e., bread, cookies) with one hand and without dropping the food or any part of it.

5. Meat Cutting: (1) Separation of the meat with the fork held in one hand, by the handle, side ways, and the meat separated by the lower side of the fork. (2) Separation of the meat with the knife held right side up, by the handle in one hand and the fork in the other with the use of the knife for cutting and the fork for holding.

6. Napkin response: Movement of the napkin to wipe food off the resident, a utensil, the table, or place in the lap.

7. Drooling: Food being removed from the mouth without being placed in a spoon (i.e., dripping pudding from the mouth, removing chewed meat from mouth into hand).

8. Licking: Licking food from any other item other than lips (e.g. licking fingers, plate, table, etc.)

9. Oversized bites: Overfilling mouth with food which prohibits chewing with the mouth closed.

10. Touching food: Any contact between hands and food that was not a self-feeding response (e.g., shoveling food onto fork with fingers, patting Jello with hands).

11. Eating too fast: Less than one-half the time allotted for eating.

12. Eating too slow: Taking more than the allotted time to eat.

13. Sitting improperly: Sits other than with back straight and feet straight down or directly on the floor.

14. Chews improperly: Swallows food almost whole, gulps food down.

15. Plays with food: Stirs food up, put hands in the middle of it and pats or squeezes it, etc.

16. Inappropriate Behavior (tantrum).

A. Screaming, yelling, hollering.

B. Hitting, slapping, or kicking.

C. Spitting.

D. Biting self or others.

E. Throwing objects.

F. Abuse to property.

G. Verbal abuse toward others.

H. Physical abuse towards self and others.

I. Removing clothing.

J. Scratching self or others.

K. Using inappropriate cuss words and sexual expressions.

CHAPTER SIX

GROOMING PROGRAM
MODEL LESSON PLANS
TABLE OF CONTENTS

Grooming Skills/Personal Appearance Evaluation

Resident _____No._____Date_____

Evaluator_____Room_____

RATING:

1. Never been observed to perform the skill by him or herself, even though he or she has had the opportunity.

2. Peforms task at times by him or herself, but not adequately (sloppy, because he or she does not know how._This means that you, the evaluator, has never seen him or her do it correctly at least once, but he or she tries.

3. Performs the task adequately with verbal prompts/assistance (if someone tells him or her to do it or how to do it).

4. Does the task, sometimes by him or herself, but not adequately (sloppy, but he or she does know how). This means that you, the evaluator, have seen him or her do it correctly at least once.

5. Performs the task adequately and consistently (most of the time) without verbal or physical assistance.

No - No opportunity to perform the task.

PD - Does not perform task due to physical/mental disability.

SKILL	RATING 1 - 5
1. Brushes or combs hair	_____
2. Sets and rolls hair	_____
3. Bathes or showers self	_____
4. Washes hands at sink	_____
5. Washes face at sink	_____
6. Dries hands or face	_____
7. Shaves face (males) with safety electric razor	_____
8. Shaves underarms (females) with safety/electric razor	_____
9. Shaves legs (females) with safety/electric razor	_____
10. Applies deodorant underarms	_____
11. Applies cosmetics (male) aftershave, lotion, powder.	_____
12. Applies cosmetics (female)	_____
A. foundation (makeup)	_____
B. lipstick	_____
C. powder	_____
D. eyebrow pencil	_____
E. perfume or cologne	_____
F. mascara	_____
13. Trims and cleans nails	_____
14. Blows nose with handkerchief	_____

15. Brushes teeth with toothbrush
and toothpaste   _____

16. Cleans mouth with mouthwash   _____

17. Washes hair with shampoo   _____

18. Washes hair with soap   _____

19. Shines shoes   _____

20. Walking   _____

     A. with head up   _____

     B. with back straight   _____

     C. with stomach in   _____

     D. with toes forward   _____

     E. with feet spaced properly   _____

     F. lifts feet off ground -
doesn't drag feet   _____

     G. walks without bouncing or
shuffling feet   _____

21. Sitting   _____

A. with legs together or
crossed (female)   _____

B. back straight   _____

C. does not sprawl   _____

22. Cares for menstrual needs
(uses sanitary devices)   _____

MODEL LESSON 200
TASK: MOUTHWASHING

GOAL: Improve grooming skills.

OBJECTIVE: To teach the resident to rinse his or her mouth with water or mouthwash and wipe his or her mouth without assistance. To be taught as a prerequisite to or simultaneously with tooth brushing.

MATERIALS: Two (2) small glasses or paper cups, a box of tissues or two (2) cloth towels.

SETTING: The resident and trainer stand at sink, facing each other.

PRE-TEST/POST-TEST: Begin with glass and tissue or towel within the resident's reach. (See notes 1, 2, and 3). The trainer touches the glass, tissue or towel and says, "John or Jane, wash your mouth". Do not reinforce a correct response and do not correct an incorrect response. Give no assistance.

TEACHING PROCEDURE

STEP 1: Begin with two (2) glasses and towels within the resident's reach. The trainer touches the towel and says, "John/Jane, wash your mouth", and immediately picks up one of the towels or tissues, wipes his or her mouth, and puts down the tissue or towel.

STEP 2: Demonstration: Begin with two (2) glasses and towels within the resident's reach. The trainer then says, "John/Jane wash your mouth", and immediately (a) picks up glass of water, (b) rinses his or her mouth, (c) spits into sink, and (d) puts down the glass.

STEP 3: Terminal Behavior: Begin with glass, towel or tissue within the resident's reach. The trainer says, "John/Jane, wash your mouth". Give minimal reinforcement and assistance as required.

NOTE 1: If the resident does not know how to turn the water on and to fill his or her glass, he or she should be taught to do so. This may be taught as a separate skill or simultaneously with the mouth washing activity if it does not become too difficult to the resident.

NOTE 2: If the resident swallows the water instead of rinsing his or her mouth, the trainer should demonstrate again, this time spitting out the water as seen as it enters his or her mouth, without rinsing. (The trainer may have to grasp the resident's jaw and gently force it open to prevent the resident's swallowing the water). Then, after the resident has mastered this, the resident can be reinforced for keeping the water in his or her mouth and rinsing without swallowing.

NOTE 3: After the resident has been taught to rinse and wipe his or her mouth, a commercial mouthwash may be introduced to the resident. The trainer should reinforce the resident when he or she uses the mouthwash appropriately.

MODEL LESSON 201
TASK: BRUSHING TEETH

GOAL: Improve grooming skills.

OBJECTIVE: To teach the resident to put toothpaste on toothbrush and to brush his or her teeth without assistance.

MATERIALS: A toothbrush appropriate in size for the resident; with small tube of toothpaste. Coordinate this lesson with mouth washing by having a glass and towel nearby in the appropriate stage.

SETTING: The resident and trainer stand at a sink, facing a mirror.

PRE-TEST/POST-TEST: Begin with toothbrush, toothpaste and glass within the resident's reach. The trainer touches the toothbrush and says, "John/Jane, brush your teeth". (See note 1). Do not reinforce a correct response and do not correct an incorrect response. Give no assistance.

TEACHING PROCEDURE

STEP 1: Begin with a toothbrush with a small amount of toothpaste on it. The trainer stands besides the resident on his right side with his or her left arm behind the resident's back and holding his or her chin with his or her left hand. The trainer (a) places the handle of the toothbrush in the resident's right hand (if he or she is right handed) and, holding the resident's right hand, (b) brings it up and places it between the resident's lips and positions it against his or her front teeth. (See note 1). The trainer says, "John/Jane, brush your teeth", and immediately moves the resident's hand up and down with the toothbrush across the front teeth. (See note 2).

STEP 2: Begin as in Step 1, the trainer tells the resident to brush his or her teeth. The resident must then brush his or her front teeth as in step 1. The trainer then says, "John/Jane, brush your teeth", and immediately physically guides the resident to move the toothbrush (which is still in his or her mouth) up and down and across the resident's teeth, brushing continually further from the center of the mouth to the right and to the left.

STEP 3: Begin as in Step 2. The trainer tells the resident to brush his or her teeth. As soon as the resident has successfully brushed the front teeth in sequence (with social reinforcement) the trainer says, "John/Jane, brush your teeth", and immediately manually guides the resident to place the toothbrush (still in the resident's hand or mouth) against the lower biting surface of the teeth and prompts the resident to brush these surfaces using physical guidance as described is Step 2.

STEP 4: Begin as in Step 2. The trainer tells the resident to brush his or her teeth. As soon as the resident has successfully brushed the front teeth, right and left of front teeth, and lower biting surface in sequence, (with social reinforcement), then the trainer says, "John/Jane, brush your teeth", and immediately places the toothbrush (in the resident's hand and already in his mouth) against the upper biting surfaces and brushes these surfaces using physical guidance as described in Step 2.

STEP 5: Begin as in Step 2. The trainer tells the resident to brush his or her teeth. As soon as the resident has successfully brushed the front teeth, right and left of the front teeth, lower biting surface, in sequence (with social reinforcement). The trainer says, "John/Jane, brush your teeth", then the trainer immediately places the toothbrush (in the resident's hand and already in his or her mouth) against the backside of lower teeth and brushes the entire area using physical guidance. Repeat similar action for the backside of the upper teeth and brushes the entire area using physical guidance.

STEP 6: The trainer places the toothpaste on it in the resident's hand and positions it in his or her mouth as in Step 1. The trainer tells the resident to brush his or her teeth. The resident should brush his or her teeth. The resident should brush his or her teeth completely. Then the trainer says, "John/Jane, brush your teeth", and using physical guidance, the trainer takes the resident's hand and brings the toothbrush down to rest under running water, rinsing it thoroughly and putting it down on the sink (or designated place). The trainer then says, "John/Jane, wash your mouth", (see note 3). The resident should wash and wipe his or her mouth. Give minimal assistance as required.

STEP 7: Begin with loaded toothbrush in the resident's hand with his or her arm outstretched with hand near faucet. Then the trainer says, "John/Jane, brush your teeth", and immediately physically guides the resident by standing behind him or her putting his or her left hand over the resident's hand and moving it towards the resident's mouth to the position described in Step 1. The resident should then perform previously learned sequence, including rinsing and wiping mouth.

STEP 8: Begin with open tube of toothpaste in the resident's left hand and brush in right hand. The trainer says, "John/Jane, brush your teeth", and immediately grasps the resident's hands and assists him or her to squeeze toothpaste on the brush. This is accomplished by the trainer holding his or her hand over the resident's hand on the toothpaste. The trainer then moves his or hand to gently squeeze the toothpaste onto the brush which is held just beneath the toothpaste tube.

STEP 9: Begin with the toothpaste with the cap removed, lying on the sink. The toothbrush is in the resident's hand. The trainer then says, "John/Jane, brush your teeth", and immediately manually guides the resident to pick up the toothpaste and position it as in Step 6. The resident should then complete brushing.

STEP 10: Begin with toothpaste with cap on the tube lying on the sink. The toothbrush is also lying on the sink alongside the toothpaste. The trainer says. "John/Jane, brush your teeth", and immediately manually guides the resident to: a) pick up the toothpaste

b) take off the cap of tube

c) pick up the toothbrush

d) align the toothbrush and paste as in Step 10. The resident should then complete brushing.

STEP 11: Begin as in Step 10. The trainer then says, "John/Jane, brush your teeth", once the resident has completed brushing his or her teeth the trainer immediately takes the resident's hand and guides him or her to pick up the toothpaste, put the cap on, pick up the brush, and put them in designated place.

NOTE 1: If the resident's teeth are not together, the trainer can gently push upward on the chin to put them together; if the resident's mouth does not open, the trainer may hold the resident's head steady with one hand and gently apply pressure on the chin in such a manner to cause him or her to open mouth.

NOTE 2: Manually guide the resident's desired movements being the least intrusive as possible in order to keep him or her from causing any physical pain, reduce the pressure immediately as the resident begins to perform the movement on his or her own. If the desired movement slows down or stops, immediately reapply just enough pressure to restore the movement. Physical guidance should continue on a given trial until the teeth have been brushed clean. It will be up to the trainer and his or her judgment as to whether on a given trial the resident has brushed long enough to have cleaned the teeth in question.

NOTE 3: In the beginning, the trainer should give the command, "John/Jane, wash your mouth", but gradually stop giving this command so that the resident performs this behavior in response to the command, "brush your teeth".

MODEL LESSON 202
TASK: HANDWASHING

GOAL: Improving grooming skills.

OBJECTIVE: To teach the resident to wash his hands upon request.

PREREQUISITE SKILLS: Upon request, the resident responds by touching his hand.

MATERIALS: Two (2) small (hotel-size) bars of soap; two (2) hand towels.

SETTING: The resident and trainer standing at a sink, facing a mirror.

PRE-TEST/POST-TEST: Begin with soap and hand towel within the resident's reach. The trainer touches the soap and says, "John, wash your hands". (See note 1). Do not reinforce a correct response and do not correct an incorrect response. Give no assistance.

TEACHING PROCEDURE

STEP 1: Begin with 2 hand towels within the resident's reach. Then the trainer says, "John, wash your hands", and immediately (a) picks up a towel and puts it between the palms of his hands, (b) holds the towel with his left hand and rubs right palm and then holds towel with his right hand and rubs left palm, until palms are dry, (c) slides the towel over the back of one hand and rubs until it is dry, then repeats this procedure with the other hand and (d) puts down the towel.

STEP 2: Begin as in Step 1. The trainer turns on the faucet in the sink. (See note 2). Then the trainer says, "John wash your hands", and immediately (a) puts his hands under the running water, (b) thoroughly rinses his hands, (c) turns off the water, and (d) dries his hands.

STEP 3: Begin with two (2) bars of soap and two (2) hand towels within the resident's reach. Then the trainer turns on the faucet in the sink. The trainer says, "John, wash your hands", and immediately (a) picks up the soap and puts it between cupped palms of his hand, (b) puts his hands under water, (c) slides his palms back and forth until lather forms, (d) puts soap down and (e) lathers back of each hand with the opposite palm.

STEP 4: The trainer says, "John, wash your hands, and immediately (a) turns water on, (b) performs above Step 3 actions in sequence and (c) thoroughly rinses his hands, turns water off and dries his hands.

STEP 6: Terminal Behavior:

Begin with soap and hand towel within the resident's reach. The trainer touches the soap and says, "John, wash our hands". Give minimal reinforcement as required.

NOTE 1: In the pre-test, post-test, and terminal behavior stages, the trainer must use his or her judgment to determine whether the resident can wash his hands sufficiently well enough to pass the criterion. However, the resident should be able to at least lather soap into the palms and to the back of both hands.

NOTE 2: The trainer should insure that the water used is not too hot. If there is only one(1) faucet, the trainer should require the hot water so that warm water runs out; if there are two (2) faucets, the trainer should plug up the sink and fill it with warm water. In the latter case, the lesson plan will need to be modified as necessary as the resident must dip hands in the water, rather than putting them under the faucet.

MODEL LESSON 203
TASK: BATHING

GOAL: Improve grooming skills.

OBJECTIVE: To teach the resident to shower, to wash all parts of his body.

MATERIALS: Soap, washcloth (see note 1), bathing suit or rain gear for the trainer.

SETTING: The resident and trainer are in the shower room, with warm water running.

PRE-TEST/ POST-TEST: Refer to "bathing checklist". The trainer hands the resident a washcloth and soap and says, "John, wash yourself". Give no assistance. Do not correct an incorrect response or reinforce a correct response. Enter on the checklist provided each part of the body washed by the resident, if any.

TEACHING PROCEDURE

STEP 1: Soaping washcloth. (See note 1). The trainer stands close to the resident while the resident is in the warm running shower. The trainer guides the resident's dominant hand to pick up the soap, and the other hand to pick up the washcloth. The trainer says, "John, wash yourself", and immediately assists the resident by grasping the resident's hands, rubbing the soap back and forth over the washcloth (see note 3).

STEP 2: Washing feet. Begin by leaning the resident over so he can touch his feet. The trainer says, "John, wash yourself", and immediately grasps the resident's hand and guides the resident to rub the cloth back and forth over the top of one foot, and then the other foot.

STEP 3: Washing lower leg. Begin as in Step 2. The trainer says, "John, wash yourself", and immediately grasps the resident's hand and guides him to rub the soaped cloth up and down (around) the lower portion of one leg, and then the other.

STEP 4: Washing upper leg or thigh. Begin by leaning the resident over slightly. The trainer then says, "John, wash_yourself", and immediately grasps the resident's hand and guides him to wash one upper leg or thigh, and then the other.

STEP 5: Washing the genital area and lower abdomen. Begin as in Step 4. The trainer then touches the resident's lower abdomen and says, "John, wash_yourself", and immediately grasps the resident's hand and guides him to wash his genitals, including the prepuce or uncircumcised area and lower abdomen.

STEP 6: Washing the rectal area and buttocks. Begin with the resident's hand, with cloth, on his hip. The trainer then says, "John, wash yourself", and immediately grasps the resident's hand and moves it around toward his back, guiding the resident to wash one buttock, then the rectal area, then the other buttock.

STEP 7: Washing the chest, stomach, and underarms. Begin by placing the resident's hand with soaped cloth on his stomach, to one side. The trainer says, "John, wash yourself", and immediately guides the resident to rub the soaped cloth up and down his side, up to his underarms, moving across, still rubbing up and down, to the other side, in the same manner.

STEP 8: Washing the arms. Begin by placing the resident's hand with soaped cloth on the back of his hand. The trainer says, "John, wash yourself", and immediately guides the resident's hand to rub the cloth up and down, and around the entire length of one arm, and then the other.

STEP 9: Washing the neck. Begin by placing the resident's hand with soaped cloth at the base of the neck. The trainer says, "John, wash yourself", and immediately guides the resident to wash around his neck, including the back of the neck.

STEP 10: Washing the face, forehead, and ears. Begin with the resident's hand with clean unused soaped cloth on the side of the face below one ear.

The trainer says, "John, wash yourself", and immediately guides the resident's hand to wash one side of his face, including the ear, moving up and down and across to the other side of the face, ending up by washing the other ear, and then the forehead.

STEP 11: Terminal Behavior. Begin with the resident in the shower. The trainer points to the soap and cloth and says, "John, wash yourself". Write down on the checklist those parts of the body the resident washes. To pass bathing, the resident should wash his entire body on three (3) separate occasions. The resident does not have to do it in the same order that he or she was taught, however, any order will do. If the resident misses a part of the body, demonstrate the washing of that part again before giving a new post-test.

NOTE 1: The mitten-washcloth will consist of two (2) washcloths sewn together at the edges and through the cloths so that the thumb and fingers are separated as with a mitten.

NOTE 2: In each demonstration step, as the trainer physically guides the resident to accomplish the task, the resident is given liberal verbal praise: "Good boy" or "Good girl", "John or Jane, you're washing yourself".

NOTE 3: When the resident has learned this lesson, it might be a good idea to train him or her to switch the cloth to the opposite hand and soap the cloth with the other hand.

MODEL LESSON 204
TASK: HAIR BRUSHING
(MODELLED)

GOAL: Improve grooming skills.

OBJECTIVE: To teach the resident to brush his/her hair upon request. (Parting the hair is not required).

PREREQUISITE SKILLS: Upon request, the resident responds by touching his or her "hair".

MATERIALS: Two light -weight small-sized brushes with handles.

SETTING: The resident and trainer are standing, facing a mirror.

PRE-TEST/ POST-TEST: Begin with a brush within the resident's reach. The trainer touches the brush and says, "John/Jane, brush your hair". (See note 1). Do not reinforce a correct response and do not correct an incorrect response. Give no assistance.

TEACHING PROCEDURE

Step 1: Begin with two brushes within the resident's reach. The trainer places a brush appropriately (with bristles facing the resident's body) in the resident's right hand. (See note 2). The trainer holds the brush in his/her right hand and says, "John/Jane, brush your hair", and immediately brushes the right side of his/her hair, beginning at the top of the head and going down to the ends of the hair. (See note 3).

STEP 2: Begin as in Step 1, with the trainer and resident holding the brushes appropriately. Then the trainer says, "John/Jane, brush your hair", and immediately brushes left side of his/her hair (crossing his/her right hand in front of his/her body), beginning at the top of his/her head and going down to the ends of his/her hair.

STEP 3: Begin as in Step 1, with the trainer and resident holding the brushes appropriately. The trainer then says, "John/Jane, brush your hair", and immediately brushes the front of his/her hair, beginning at the top of his/her head and going forward to the ends of his/her hair.

STEP 4: Begin as in Step 1, with the trainer and resident holding the brushes appropriately. The trainer says, "John/Jane, brush your hair", and immediately brushes the back of his/her hair, beginning at the top of his/her head and going backwards to the ends of his/her hair.

STEP 5: Begin with two brushes within the resident's reach. The trainer then says, "John/Jane, brush your hair", and immediately (a) picks up the brush and holds it appropriately, (b) brushes sides, front, and back of his/her hair in any order, and (c) puts the brush down. The trainer may need to give his/her additional cues in order for the resident to complete the entire sequence of actions by pointing to a part of the resident's hair that has not been brushed.

STEP 6: Terminal Behavior. Begin with the brush within the resident's reach. The trainer touches the brush and says, "John/Jane, brush your hair". Give minimal reinforcement and assistance as required.

NOTE 1: In the past, terminal behavior and post-test stages, the trainer must use his/ her judgment to determine whether the resident can brush his/her hair sufficiently well enough to pass criterion. The resident should be able to leave his/her hair somewhat smooth, (depending on the texture, thickness, and curl of the resident's hair) and in orderly fashion.

NOTE 2: This lesson plan is written for a right - handed resident. If the resident is left-handed, the trainer should make the appropriate revisions in the lesson plan.

NOTE 3: Where on top of the head the resident begins to brush depends on where the resident's hair is parted. Also, depending on the resident's hair style, the resident may need to be taught to brush (1) side hair back behind his/her ears, rather than straight down, or (2) front hair back to the top of the head, rather than forward.

MODEL LESSON 205
TASK - NOSE BLOWING

GOAL: Improve grooming skills.

OBJECTIVE: To teach the resident to blow his/her nose upon request.

PREREQUISITE SKILLS: Upon request the resident responds by touching "nose".

MATERIALS: A box of tissues and a wastebasket.

SETTING: The resident and trainer standing or sitting.

PRE-TEST/POST-TEST: Begin with tissue and wastebasket within the reach of the resident. The trainer touches the tissue and says, "John/Jane, blow your nose". (See note 1). Do not reinforce a correct response and do not correct an incorrect response. Give no assistance.

STEP 1: Begin with tissue and wastebasket within the resident's reach. The trainer then says, "John/Jane, blow your nose", and immediately, (a) picks up a tissue, (b) places the tissue under his/her nose and wipes his/her nose using his/her thumb and forefinger, and (c) puts the tissue into the wastebasket.

STEP 2: Begin as in Step 1. The trainer then says, "John/Jane, blow your nose", and immediately, (a) picks up a tissue, (b) places tissue under his/her nose, (c) blows hard through his/her nasal cavity so that there is audible sound, and (d) wipes his/her nose and puts tissue into wastebasket. (See note 2).

STEP 3: Terminal Behavior. Begin with tissue and wastebasket within the resident's reach. The trainer touches the tissue and says, "John/Jane, blow your nose". Give minimal reinforcement and assistance as required.

NOTE 1: In the pre-test, the terminal behavior and post-test steps, the trainer must use his/her judgment to determine whether the resident can blow his/her nose sufficiently well enough to pass criterion. The resident should be able to at least to blow through his/her nasal cavity and wipe his/her nose with a tissue.

NOTE 2: If the resident has difficulty blowing through his/her nose and/or nasal cavity (many individuals persist in blowing through their mouths), the trainer should place his/her hand over the resident's mouth so that the air will have to come through their nose. However, the resident should not be taught to close his/her mouth when blowing his/her nose, because this can cause permanent damage to the ear drums.

MODEL LESSON 206
TASK: SHAVING WITH SAFETY RAZOR

GOAL: Improve grooming skills.

OBJECTIVE: To teach the resident to shave his face with a safety razor, without assistance.

PREREQUISITE SKILLS: To touch face with hand safety razor without blade.

MATERIALS: Two (2) safety razors, single - edged blades, can of shaving cream.

SETTING: The resident and trainer in bathroom in front of a mirror which is hanging over a sink.

PRE-TEST/POST-TEST: Begin with shaving cream, and safety razor within the resident's reach. The trainer touches (a) shaving cream and (b) safety razor and says, "John, shave your beard". Do not reinforce a correct response and do not correct an incorrect response. Give no assistance.

TEACHING PROCEDURE

STEP 1: The trainer and resident stand in front of the sink. All materials for shaving are within the resident's reach. The trainer says, "John, shave your beard", and immediately the trainer models (a) turning on the water, (b) adjusting the temperature of water and (c) wetting the face and neck areas, then, the resident is expected to imitate the modeling of the trainer.

STEP 2: Begin as in conditions in Step 1. The trainer says, "John, shave your beard", and immediately the trainer models (a) picking up shaving cream and shaking the can several times, (b) pushing the bottom to top of the can of shaving cream, and (3) aiming shaving cream into free hand, then the resident is expected to imitate the modelling of the trainer.

STEP 3: Begin with shaving cream in hand of resident. The trainer then says, "John, shave your beard", and immediately the trainer models (a) applying shaving cream to one side of his face, beginning at the bottom of his sideburn, and continuing downward to his chin, (b) then apply cream to the other side of the face down to the chin, (c) covering the area beneath the chin, and each side of neck to be shaved, d) covering the upper and lower lip and (e) rinsing hands in the wash basin. The resident is expected to imitate the modelling of the trainer.

STEP 4: Begin with the beard area covered with shaving cream. (See Note 1). "John, shave your beard", and immediately the trainer models (a) picking up and holding the razor against face, just below sideburn. The trainer will shave down one side - repeating the motion on two occasions. (b) The trainer rinses the razor and (c) the trainer shaves any other unshaved area or that side of the face - repeating the motion two times. The trainer rinses razor.

STEP 5: Begin with the beard area covered with shaving cream. The trainer performs the tasks listed in Step 4, and then the trainer models (a) shaving the opposite side of the face, beginning at the bottom edge of sideburn. The trainer shaves down one side, repeating this motion twice. (b) The trainer rinses razor, and (c) the trainer shaves unshaven portion of cheek as before, repeating the motion twice. The trainer rinses razor.

STEP 6: Begin with beard area covered with shaving cream. The trainer models all previously learned behaviors of Steps 4 and 5. The trainer then models shaving upper lip, using a downward stroke. The trainer rinses razor.

STEP 7: The trainer models all the behaviors in Steps 4 through 6, and then models: shaving the neck using either an upward or downward stroke, as necessary. The trainer then rinses razor.

STEP 8: Begin with terminal condition of face as in Step 4. For later trials on the same day, put soap on face. The trainer says, "John, shave your beard", and immediately the trainer models:

(A) Placing hands under faucet, while other hand turns on the cold water.

(B) Also putting the free hand under faucet and forming a cup with his hands, such that water is contained in the cup.

(C) Splashing the water up against his face and wiping neck and face area, until free of leftover shaving cream.

(D) Turns off water.

(E) Takes a towel and dries face and neck. The resident is expected to imitate.

MODEL LESSON 207
TASK: SHAVING WITH ELECTRIC RAZOR

GOAL: Improve grooming skills.

OBJECTIVE: To teach the resident to shave his beard with an electric razor without assistance.

MATERIALS: Electric razor.

SETTINGS: The resident and trainer in front of mirror.

PRETEST/POST-TEST: Begin with electric razor within reach of resident. The trainer touches the electric razor and says, "John, shave your beard". Do not reinforce a correct response and do not correct an incorrect response. Give no assistance.

TEACHING PROCEDURE

STEP 1: The trainer and resident stand in front of the mirror. All materials for shaving are nearby. The trainer says, "John, shave your beard", and immediately the trainer models:

(a) Picking up and holding the razor correctly,

(b) Picking up the cord and plugging it into electrical outlet,

(c) Push starter button to turn the razor on,

(d) Placing razor against face, just below sideburn. The trainer will shave one side, repeating the motion until shaving area is free of facial hair.

(e) The trainer will share any other unshaved area on that side of face, repeating the motion until shaving area is free of facial hair.

STEP 2: Begin by performing tasks listed in Step 1. The trainer models (a) shaving the opposite side of face, beginning at the bottom edge of sideburn. The trainer shaves down one side, repeating the motions until the shaving area is free of facial hair. (b) The trainer shaves unshaved portion of cheek as before, repeating the motions until the unshaved area is free of facial hair.

STEP 3: Begin by the trainer modeling all previous behaviors in Steps 1 through 2. Then, the trainer models shaving the upper lip.

STEP 4: Begin by the trainer modeling all previous behaviors in Steps 1 through 3 and then the trainer models shaving the neck, lower lip, and chin using either an upward, downward or a combination of both until unshaved area is free of facial hair.

STEP 5: Terminal Behavior. Begin with terminal conditions of Step 4, the trainer says, "John, shave your beard". The resident is expected to imitate.

COMMENT: After it has been determined that the resident can shave himself, require him to be clean shaven everyday, i.e., reinforce him periodically during the day for being clean shaven.

MODEL LESSON 208
TASK: PICKING HAIR

OBJECTIVE: To teach the resident to pick her hair upon request.

PREREQUISITE SKILLS: Upon request, the resident responds by touching hair.

MATERIALS: One hair pick with handle.

PRE-TEST/POST-TEST: Begin with hair pick within the resident's reach. The trainer touches the hair pick and says, "Jane, pick your hair". Do not reinforce a correct response and do not correct an incorrect response. Give no assistance.

TEACHING PROCEDURE

STEP 1: The trainer says, "Jane, pick your hair", and immediately assists the resident to take hands, (a) pat left side of hair with left hand and pat right side of hair with right hand, simultaneously, (b) then, pat hair moving toward back until fingers meet.

STEP 2: Begin as in Step 1, with the trainers hand over the resident's and the trainer says, "Jane, pick your hair", and immediately assists the resident to pat front of hair (using both hands) moving backward until back hairline is reached.

STEP 3: Begin with hair pick within the resident's reach. The trainer places the hair pick appropriately in the resident's right hand. The trainer places her right hand over the resident's right hand and says, "Jane, pick your hair", and immediately assists the resident to hold the hair pick in preferred hand and (a) pushing pick back inserting in hair at front hair line, (b) and then pulling the hair upward and out of hair.

STEP 4: Begin as in Step 3, with the resident holding the pick appropriately in right hand with the trainer's hand over the resident's, the trainer says, "Jane, pick your hair", and immediately assists the resident to (a) insert the hair pick in the hair at right hairline (above ear), (b) and then pulling the hair pick upward and out of hair. This is continued moving toward the back along the hairline.

STEP 5: Begin as in Step 4, with the resident holding the hair pick appropriately in dominant hand with the trainer's hand over the resident's, the trainer says, "Jane, pick your hair", and immediately assists the resident to (a) insert the hair pick in hair left hairline (above ear) (b) and then pulling pick upward and out of hair. This is continued moving toward the back along the hairline.

STEP 6: Begin as in Step 5 with the resident holding the hair-pick appropriately in the preferred hand with the trainer's head over the residents. The trainer says, "Jane, pick your hair", and immediately assists the resident to (a) pick into the hair at back hair-line, (b) and then pull the hair pick upward and out of hair. This continues moving toward the top of the head.

STEP 7: Begin with hair pick in the resident's reach. The trainer says, "Jane, pick your hair", and immediately assists the resident to (a) pick up the hair pick and hold it appropriately in preferred hand, (b) pick hair front, and back and on both sides (in any order). The trainer may need to give additional cues in the task request for the resident to complete the entire sequence of actions by pointing to a part of the resident's hair that has not been picked.

CHAPTER SEVEN

SELF-HELP PROGRAMS (ADL'S)

TABLE OF CONTENTS

MODEL LESSON 300
TASK: BED MAKING

OBJECTIVE: To teach the resident to make a bed properly without assistance.

MATERIALS: A bed with two (2) sheets, a pillow and a spread.

SETTING: In bedroom, the trainer and resident standing in a position to make a bed.

PRE-TEST/POST-TEST: The trainer puts bed making materials on the bed, and points to materials, and says, "John, make up your bed". Do not reinforce a correct response and do not correct an incorrect response. Give no assistance. The trainer must use his or her judgment to determine whether the resident has completely made up the bed properly.

TEACHING PROCEDURE

For each training step the trainer will begin with the bed completely made up to the step required for training for that particular stage. The trainer will then model the behavior required at the step in the stage for the resident to imitate, giving assistance in the task request when it is needed.

FORWARD CHAINING SEQUENCE
FOR TRAINER'S USE

1. Place the bottom sheet on the bed.

2. Straighten and smooth out the bottom sheet.

3. Tuck in the bottom sheet on the sides, head and foot of the bed.

4. Miter the corners of the bottom sheet at the head and foot of the bed.

5. Place the top sheet on the bottom sheet on the bed.

6. Straighten and smooth the top sheet.

7. Place the spread on top of the sheet on the bed.

8. Straighten and smooth out the spread.

9. Tuck the spread and top sheet in at the foot of the bed (single operation).

10. Miter the corners of the spread and top sheet at the foot of the bed (single operation).

11. Pull the top sheet to the head of the bed and smooth it out.

12. Place the pillow on the top sheet at the head of the bed.

13. Pull the spread up over the pillow, straighten and smooth it out around the pillow.

BACKWARD TRAINING SEQUENCE FOR TRAINING

STEP 1: Pulling bedspread over the pillow and smoothing it out.

STEP 2: Laying the pillow at the head of the bed.

STEP 3: Pulling the top of the sheet to the head of the bed.

STEP 4: Mitering the corners of the spread and the top sheet at the foot of the bed.

STEP 5: Tucking the spread and the top sheet in at the foot of the bed.

STEP 6: Straightening and smoothing out the spread.

STEP 7: Placing the spread on the bed.

STEP 8: Straightening and smoothing out the spread.

STEP 9: Placing the top sheet on the bed.

STEP 10: Mitering the corners of the bottom sheet at the head of the bed.

STEP 11: Tucking in the bottom sheet around the mattress.

STEP 12: Straightening and smoothing out the bottom sheet.

STEP 13: Placing the bottom sheet on the bed.

MODEL LESSON 301
TASK: SWEEPING

OBJECTIVE: To teach the resident to sweep dirt into a dustpan and deposit it into a wastebasket.

MATERIALS: A broom, wastebasket, dustpan, and pieces of paper/cloth scraps.

SETTING: As required for each step.

PRE-TEST/POST-TEST: Begin with crumpled paper on the floor (or pieces of cloth), place the dustpan approximately six (6) inches away. And the trainer says, "John, sweep the floor". Give no assistance. Do not reinforce a correct response.

TEACHING PROCEDURE

The following sequence will be used to teach sweeping. Each step will involve the trainer demonstrating the sequence up to the task required for a given step. The trainer will withdraw assistance in the task request so that resident can complete that step and previously learned steps by himself.

FORWARD CHAINING SEQUENCE

STEP 1: Take one-quarter of a sheet of paper, or cloth, and crumple it into a ball and place it on the floor.

STEP 2: Place the dustpan on the floor facing the paper or scraps of cloth, approximately six (6) inches from the material.

STEP 3: Place the wastebasket two (2) to three (3) feet from the dustpan.

STEP 4: Say to the resident. "John, sweep the floor".

STEP 5: Take the broom, stand behind the resident and place the broom into his hands, however, the trainer also holds the broom herself with her arms around the resident (as in golf).

STEP 6: Sweep the material into the dustpan as the resident holds the broom.

STEP 7: The trainer and the resident lay down the broom.

STEP 8: Pick up the dustpan, tilt the dustpan backward towards the body so that the material will not fall out.

STEPS FOR TRAINING

STEP 1: The trainer completes the sequence up to emptying the contents in the dustpan into the wastebasket.

STEP 2: The trainer completes the sequence up to laying down the broom.

STEP 3: The trainer completes the sequence up to sweeping the material into the dustpan.

STEP 4: The trainer repeats Step 3, gradually extending the wastebasket away from the dustpan.

STEP 5: The trainer completes the sequence up to picking up the broom.

STEP 6: The trainer completes step five (5), but add a greater amount of smaller pieces of paper/cloth/material on the floor.

STEP 7: The trainer repeats Step 5, but puts regular type of household debris on the floor, with dustpan placed increasingly farther away from the material.

IRONING PROGRAM

OBJECTIVE: To teach the resident to iron his clothing so that he may meet community and social standards for personal appearance and self-sufficiently.

MATERIALS: An iron, ironing board with cover, water sprayer, (steam iron or teach the resident to wet clothing by dropping water from fingers) and spray starch if available.

TEACHING PROCEDURE

Modelling procedure will be used for this program. This means that the trainer will demonstrate each step by actually doing it him or herself. The trainer will give the command, "John, iron your _____ (article of clothing), and immediately perform the desired sequence himself. If the resident does not imitate the trainer, he must be physically assisted to perform the desired behavior. If the resident does imitate the trainer's behavior, the trainer will immediately reinforce the resident and proceed to the next step in the training procedure. If at any point during the procedure the resident fails to attempt to initiate, the trainer physically assist the resident in making the response and socially reinforce him. The criterion for moving to the next step in training will be defined as correct imitation of the trainer's behavior without physical assistance. All attempts or approximations to the modelled response by the resident are to be socially reinforced by the trainer. When appropriate, edible reinforcers may also be used.

The following lesson plans for ironing are numbered according to the articles of clothing. The order in which the lesson plans are taught does not matter.

MODEL LESSON 303
TASK: IRON HANDKERCHIEF

STEP 1: Press edges smooth.

STEP 2: Press from bottom right edge in towards center in continuous strokes across entire article and back to right edge (for right - handed residents).

STEP 3: Move iron up right edge to the next un-ironed section and across entire article and back.

STEP 4: Continue in this fashion until entire article is ironed.

STEP 5: Fold article in half and lightly iron.

STEP 6: Fold once or twice if necessary and again iron over it lightly.

MODEL LESSON 304
TASK: IRON NARROW SHEET/PILLOW CASE

NOTE: (Flat articles longer, but no wider than surface of ironing board):

STEP 1: Place top edge of article along top edge of ironing board.

STEP 2: Press top edge, and as much as possible of side edges, smooth.

STEP 3: Press top edge of article along top edge of ironing board.

STEP 4: Move article up to next un-ironed section and iron as in Step 1.

STEP 5: Continue moving article up and ironing edges first, then moving it from edge towards center until article is completely ironed.

STEP 6: Fold to appropriate size and lightly press.

MODEL LESSON 305
TASK: IRON LARGE SHEET

NOTE: (Flat articles longer and wider than surface of ironing board).

STEP 1: Fold article in half.

STEP 2: Place one of narrow edges along top of ironing board.

STEP 3: Press top edge, and as much as possible of side edges, smooth.

STEP 4: Press top edge of article along top edge of board.

STEP 5: Move article up to next un-ironed section and iron as in Steps 2 and 3.

STEP 6: Continue moving article up and ironing edges first, then moving in from edge towards center until article is completely ironed.

STEP 7: Turn article to other side and proceed as above. The resident must perform Steps 3 through 6 to pass Step 7.

STEP 8: Fold to appropriate size and lightly press.

MODEL LESSON 306
TASK: IRON STRAIGHT A-LINED SKIRTS

STEP 1: Holding skirt by the hem, pull skirt onto the board so that one (1) side of skirt, by the zipper or buttons, is above the surface of the ironing board and smooth with hand.

STEP 2: Press zipper on material around buttons firmly.

STEP 3: Place iron on hem of skirt point of the iron towards waistband.

STEP 4: Make a series of movements the length of the skirt from hem to waistband back to hem turning the skirt as ironed until the entire skirt is free of wrinkles.

STEP 5: If there is a kick-pleat; smooth appropriately with hands and press.

STEP 6: Remove the skirt and three (3) or four (4) inches of the skirt below the waistband.

MODEL LESSON 307
TASK: IRON GATHERED SKIRT

STEP 1: Hold the skirt by the hem, pull the skirt onto the ironing board so that one side of the skirt by the zipper or buttons is above the surface of the ironing board and smooth with hand.

STEP 2: Press the zipper on the material around the buttons firmly.

STEP 3: Place the iron on the hem with the point of the iron towards the waistband.

STEP 4: Make a movement from the hem towards the waistband as far as the gathers, and then press between the gathers in line with the movement.

STEP 5: Turn the skirt as it is ironed until the entire article is free of wrinkles.

STEP 6: Remove the article and place it on the ironing board again, pulling the waistband on first, iron the waistband smooth.

MODEL LESSON 308
TASK: IRON SLEEVELESS BLOUSE

STEP 1: Place the blouse on narrow end of the ironing board so that the end protrudes from armhole and shoulders seam up; iron shoulder seam and as much of the blouse as possible (include sleeve edge or front section).

STEP 2: Switch the blouse so as the end of the ironing board protrudes from the other armhole and repeat Step 1.

STEP 3: If the blouse has a yoke, place it smoothly on the ironing board and iron.

STEP 4: Place one front section of the blouse with buttons on the ironing board.

STEP 5: Iron the edge around the buttons and entire front section.

STEP 6: Iron the sleeve edge on the front section.

STEP 7: Turn the blouse so the side seam is on the board, press as much of the sleeve edge as possible.

STEP 8: Turn the blouse to the back so as to iron the rest of the sleeve edge; iron from the button edge of the back to the yoke or to the collar whichever the case, until the entire back section is free of wrinkles, including the back of the sleeve of the other armhole.

STEP 9: Turn the blouse so the side of the seam is on the ironing board and press.

STEP 10: Turn the blouse so the other side of the seam is on the ironing board and press.

STEP 11: Place the collar on the ironing board, underneath the side up, iron and turn the collar to the top side and iron.

MODEL LESSON 309
TASK: IRON SIMPLE BLOUSE WITH SLEEVE

STEP 1: Place one of the sleeves on the ironing board, crease along the underarm seam, and smooth the sleeve and press. Special attention is given to the cuffs, iron up to the over - shoulder seam.

STEP 2: Place the blouse on the narrow end of the ironing board so that the end protrudes from the armhole and shoulder seam up; iron the shoulder seam and as much of the blouse as possible (include the sleeve edge or front section).

STEP 3: Place the other sleeve on the ironing board and repeat Step 2 above.

STEP 4: Switch the blouse so as the end of the ironing board protrudes from the other armhole and repeat Step 2.

STEP 5: If the blouse has a yoke, place it smoothly on the ironing board and iron.

STEP 6: Place one (1) front section of the blouse with button's on the ironing board.

STEP 7: Iron the edge around the buttons and the entire front section.

MODEL LESSON 310
TASK: IRON DRESS WITH A-LINE SKIRT

STEP 1: Place one (1) sleeve on the ironing board, crease is along underarm seam, smooth the seam and press. Special attention is given to the cuffs. Iron up to the over-shoulder seam.

STEP 2: Place the top of the dress on the narrow end of the ironing board so that the end protrudes from the armhole and the shoulder seam up. Iron the shoulder seam and as much of the blouse as possible (include the sleeve's edge or front section).

STEP 3: Place the other sleeve on the ironing board and repeat Step 2 above.

STEP 4: Switch the dress top so that the end of the ironing board protrudes from the other armhole and repeat Step 2.

STEP 5: If the dress top has a yoke, place it smoothly on the ironing board and iron.

STEP 6: Place one (1) front section of the dress top with button's on the ironing board.

STEP 7: Iron the edge around the button's and the entire front section.

STEP 8: Holding the dress skirt by the hem, pull the skirt onto the ironing board so that one (1) side of the skirt by the zipper or button is above the surface of the ironing board and smooth out.

STEP 9: Press the zipper on the material around the buttons firmly.

STEP 10: Place the iron on the hem of the skirt with the point of the iron towards the waistband.

STEP 11: Make a series of movements the length of the skirt from the hem to the waistband and back to the hem turning the skirt as it is ironed until the entire skirt is wrinkle free.

STEP 12: If there is a kick - pleat, smooth appropriately with hands and press.

STEP 13: Remove the skirt from the ironing board and place it on the ironing board again with waistband on first.

STEP 14: Iron the waistband three (3) or four (4) inches below the waistband.

STEP 15: If required, press the belt.

MODEL LESSON 311
TASK: IRON DRESS WITH GATHERED SLEEVE

STEP 1: Place one (1) sleeve on the ironing board, crease along the underarm seam, smooth seam and press. Special attention is given to the cuffs. Iron up to over-shoulder seam.

STEP 2: Place the top of the dress on the narrow end of the ironing board so that the end protrudes from the armhole and shoulder seam up. Iron from the armhole and shoulder seam up. Iron the shoulder seam and as much of the blouse as possible (include sleeve edge of front section).

STEP 3: Place the other sleeve on the ironing board and repeat Step 2 above.

STEP 4: Switch the dress top so that the end of the ironing board protrudes from the other armhole and repeat Step 2.

STEP 5: If the dress has a yoke, place it smoothly on the ironing board and iron.

STEP 6: Place one (1) front section of the dress top with buttons on the ironing board.

STEP 7: Iron the edge around the button's and entire front section of the dress.

STEP 8: Holding the skirt by the hem, pull the skirt onto the ironing board so that one side of the skirt by the zipper or buttons is above the surface of the ironing board and smooth with hand.

STEP 9: Press the zipper on the material around the buttons firmly.

STEP 10: Place the iron on the hem with the point of the iron towards the waistband.

STEP 11: Make a movement from the hem towards the waistband as far as the gathers, and then press between the gathers in line with the movement.

STEP 12: Turn the skirt as it is being ironed until the entire article is free of wrinkles.

STEP 13: Remove the article and place it on the ironing board again pulling the waistband on first, iron waistband smooth.

STEP 14: If needed, press the belt.

MODEL LESSON 312
TASK: IRON PANTS (JEANS OR SLACKS)

STEP 1: Pull the pants inside out (if needed).

STEP 2: Find the front left pocket and iron it flat against the inside of the pants leg. Do the same for the right pocket.

STEP 3: Pull the pants right side out.

STEP 4: Put the waist end of the pants around the ironing board so that only one layer of the waistband is lying on top of the ironing board. Pull the pants onto board as far as they will go.

STEP 5: Begin on the front right and iron from the waist of the pants inward, lifting the iron at the pocket so that it does not snag inside entrance to the pocket. Then put it down and iron the pocket smooth.

STEP 6: Adjust left front and repeat Step 5.

STEP 7: As neatly as possible, adjust the pressure on the iron and smooth over zipper flap without leaving creases in the flap.

STEP 8: Pull the pants around so that the back left side is on the top of the ironing board; i.e., seam separating the back left and front left is near inside edge of the ironing board. Iron from the waist in, inward, lifting the iron slightly to avoid snagging then put it down and iron the pocket smoothly. Iron as far inward as possible, and over the seam.

STEP 9: Continue pulling the pants around (in same direction as before) so that the back center seam is resting near the inside edge of the ironing board, and the other (right) side of the back side is ironed in the same way as the left back side.

STEP 10: Then arrange the pants where the crotch area can be ironed (can be done by pulling the top at waist outside the area of pants away from the resident and down from the ironing board). Iron as smoothly as possible using the point of the iron.

STEP 11: Pull the pants off the ironing board. Take the right leg and hold the cuff area up in the air (straight up-above the resident's waist). Take the two seams and match them together; hold them there and lay the leg on the ironing board, such that the outside seam is in the center of the leg facing up (at the same time, the inside seam is directly beneath the outside seam, and also in the center of the pants leg). Now iron over the pants leg on both sides of the outside seam, bearing down with more pressure at the long edge of the pants where it meets the ironing board, forming a crease.

STEP 12: Turn the leg over so that the inside of the leg is face up. Iron it as the outside had been done.

STEP 13: Take the right leg and iron as the left leg was done in Steps 11 and 12.

STEP 14: If the pants have cuffs on them, take the left leg and when ironing near the cuffs, lift the iron so as not to snag it, then bring the iron down on top of the cuff and iron as before. This is true for Steps 12, and 13, also.

CHAPTER EIGHT

MODEL LESSON 400

TASK: TOILET TRAINING

GOAL: Improve toileting skills.

OBJECTIVE: To teach the resident to use the toilet independently, without verbal, gestural or physical assistance and/or prompts, and to eliminate in the toilet bowl exclusive of other areas in his or her environment. This does not include wiping one's self, or flushing the toilet. These are separate training programs and should be taught later.

MATERIALS: A clock and edible reinforcement.

SETTING: The trainer and resident stands near a toilet during training. Both move further and further away from the toilet area as training progresses. Training is done approximately two (2) hours prior to bedtime. The resident is given as much beverage or water every thirty (30) minutes during his or her awake time until training begins two (2) hours prior to bedtime.

BASELINE:

STEP 1: Observe/monitor the resident and record all incidences of, i.e. time of wetting, or if his/her clothes or in toilet.

STEP 2: (Initiate beverage or water here) and record all incidences of wetting (the time and whether incident is in clothes or in toilet). In both phases, if the resident eliminates in the toilet, note whether or not, (1) he or she was taken and cared for, (2) he or she went on command, or (3) he or she went by him or herself.

Baseline Coding may be done by recording using the code below:

T- toilet

C- clothes

Ta- taken to toilet

Tc - goes to toilet on command

Ti- goes to toilet independently

Data recording: The time of wetting and whether T, C, Ta, Tc, or Ti continues daily throughout the toilet training program.

TEACHING PROCEDURE
SITTING ON COMMODE

STEP 1: Begin with the resident seated on the commode with his pants down, the trainer says, "John, go to the bathroom". The resident is rewarded by being given an edible with social praise for sitting on the commode for five (5) seconds without getting up, or without being disruptive. Once the resident performs task appropriately and has been rewarded for three (3) times in a row, proceed to Step 2.

STEP 2: Begin with the resident seated on the commode with his pants down. The trainer says, "John, go to the bathroom". The resident is rewarded with edible and with social praise for sitting on the commode for five (5) seconds without getting up, or without being disruptive. Once the resident sits on the commode for three (3) minutes without attempting to leave, proceed to Step 3.

NOTE: The idea is to extend the resident's sitting time on the commode from a few seconds (five seconds) to three (3) minutes. For example, Trial 1 might require his sitting for 7 seconds before edible and social reinforcement is given; Trial 2, 15 seconds; trial 3, 30 seconds; Trial 4, 45 seconds; Trial 5, 60 seconds; Trial 6, 2 minutes; and Trial 7, 3 minutes.

STEP 3: Begin with the resident standing in front of the commode (dressed). The trainer says, "John, go to the bathroom", the trainer takes the resident's two hands in his/her two hands and assists the resident to grasp the waistband at both sides (thumbs hooked inside the waistband, fingers outside) and pushes pants down so that the waistband is just below the resident's knees. The trainer then gives the resident social and verbal praise when the task is completed. The trainer then helps the resident sit on the commode.

Repeat the task request as needed gradually withdrawing physical assistance until the resident can perform the task independently. When the resident is able to perform the task by himself the trainer says, "John, go to the bathroom". The resident (without assistance) is expected to pull down his pants and sit on the commode. Any and all positive responses to these behaviors are rewarded with social praise plus an edible reinforcement.

ADDITIONAL TRIALS: All subsequent trials are the same and all of the assigned tasks must be carried out by the resident before he is rewarded. Be sure to leave the resident on the commode for three (3) minutes before beginning a new trial. This step continues until the resident completes the entire task independently pulling his pants down and sitting on the commode by himself.

STEP 4: (Pulling pants up)

Begin with the resident in front of the toilet (dressed) the trainer says, "John, go to the bathroom". The resident repeats Step 3, i.e., pulls down his pants and sits on the commode. The trainer stands the resident up, takes the resident's two hands in his/her two hands and assists the resident to grasp the waistband on both sides (thumbs hooked inside the waistband, fingers outside) and pulls the pants up to the waist. The trainer gives social praise ("Good boy, John - you pulled up your pants") to the resident when the task is completed.

The resident repeats the task (no physical assistance allowed).

The trainer says, "John, go to the bathroom". The resident is expected to push pants down, sit on the commode for approximately three (3) minutes and then pull pants back up. And approximation to pulling the pants back up after having sat on the commode is rewarded with edible (food) and social (praise) reinforcement.

STEP 5: SUBSEQUENT TRIALS.

More and more approach behavior must be accomplished by the resident before an award is given. This Step 5 continues until the resident approaches and goes through the sequence, ninety five percent (95%) of the trials over a four (4) day period of time. Reinforcement may be given intermittently for each of the trials in the sequence. An example of this is as follows:

TRIAL I: The resident approaches the commode and stops two (2) feet away (do not reinforce).

(a) The trainer repeats command and the resident continues towards the commode (do not reinforce).

(b) The trainer repeats command and the resident pulls pants down (reinforce).

(c) The trainer repeats command and the resident sits on the commode for approximately three (3) minutes (reinforce).

(d) The trainer repeats command and the resident pulls pants up (reinforce).

STEP 6: Approaches the commode two (2) feet and stops.

(a) No reinforcement

(b) The trainer repeats command.

(c) The resident moves away from commode or stands still.

STEP 7: The resident approaches commode three (3) feet and stops. The trainer gives reinforcement. The trainer repeats command and the resident continues walking toward the commode. The trainer gives reinforcement. The resident sits on the commode for approximately three (3) minutes. The trainer gives social reinforcement only. The resident pulls pants up, the trainer gives reinforcement.

STEP 8: The resident approaches the commode and reaches it.

(a) The trainer gives reinforcement.

(b) The resident pulls pants down.

(c) The trainer gives social reinforcement.

(d) The resident sits on the commode for one (1) minute with no elimination. The trainer gives no reinforcement.

The resident is encouraged to sit on the commode by the trainer if he or she attempts to get up from the commode.

(a) The trainer gives no reinforcement.

(b) The resident pulls down pants assisted.

(c) The trainer gives no reinforcement.

STEP 9: The resident approaches the commode and reaches it.

(a) The trainer gives reinforcement.

(b) The resident pulls pants down.

(c) The trainer gives social reinforcement.

(d) The resident sits on the commode for three (3) minutes.

(e) The trainer gives social reinforcement.

(f) The resident pulls up pants.

(g) The trainer gives reinforcement.

STEP 10: The resident approaches the commode and reaches it.

(a) The trainer gives social reinforcement.

(b) The resident pulls down pants.

(c) The trainer gives reinforcement.

(d) The resident sits on commode.

(e) The trainer gives social reinforcement.

(f) The resident pulls pants up.

(g) The trainer gives reinforcement.

STEP 11: The resident approaches the commode and reaches it.

(a) The trainer gives social reinforcement.

(b) The resident pulls pants down.

(c) The trainer does not give reinforcement.

(d) The resident sits on the commode.

(e) The trainer does not give reinforcement.

(f) The resident pulls pants up.

(g) The trainer gives social reinforcement.

Proceed to Step 6 when the resident has succeeded in completing ninety-five percent (95%) of the sequences over a period of four (4) days. Illustrated above is given reinforcement only after correct responses and fading out all reinforcement gradually. The last two (2) responses to be rewarded are the procedures the resident is trying to learn (approach behavior) and the final behavior in the sequence (pulling the pants back up).

STEP 12: (Command approach behavior continued). Begin with the resident at the bathroom door. The trainer says, "John, go to the bathroom". The resident is expected to approach the commode and pull his pants down, sit for approximately three (3) minutes and pull his pants up. Approximations to this approach are handled in same manner as in Step 5.

STEP 13: (Command approach behavior continued). Begin with the resident out of sight of commode. The trainer says, "John, go to the bathroom". The same procedure is followed as in Step 4.

STEP 14: (Command approach behavior continued). Begin with the resident in a group on the ward. Continue same procedure as in Step 4.

STEP 15: Continue same approach as done in Step 14 with the trainer saying, "John, go to the bathroom". At this step the trainer begins to fade out all reinforcements. The trainer reinforces the resident on the average of every 3rd trial.

STEP 16: Continue reinforcing the resident on every 3rd trial during the next 2 steps and begin fading out other cues. The trainer points to the bathroom, and calls the resident by name.

STEP 17: The trainer continues process and continuous fading. Someone else with whom the resident is unfamiliar points to the bathroom and tells the resident to go to the bathroom.

STEP 18: Reward the resident any and all times he or she may go to the bathroom alone independently.

STEP 19: Fade out all above steps and reinforcement slowly as resident can perform task independently.

CHAPTER NINE

MODEL LESSON 402

TASK: EYE CONTACT

OBJECTIVE: To teach the resident to attend or look at the trainer when his or her name is called.

MATERIALS: Two (2) chairs and reinforcements.

SETTING: Trainer sitting face to face with resident.

TEACHING PROCEDURE

The trainer should be directly in front of the resident close enough for the trainer to manually move the resident's head so that he or she faces him or her. The trainer should say, "John/Jane, look at me". If the resident looks at the trainer, he or she is to be reinforced immediately. If he or she does not look at the trainer, then with one hand, the trainer should turn the resident's head so that the resident is facing the trainer. With the other hand, the trainer should place the reinforcement between his or her face until the resident attends to the trainer. If the resident resists shaping, the trainer should continue the process, with minimal assistance, until the resident looks at him or her without great resistance.

REINFORCEMENT: If the resident looks at the trainer on his or her own, then the resident gets reinforced immediately. The trainer gives reinforcement after his or her completion of assisted response.

NUMBER OF TRIALS PER RESIDENT: Six (6) minutes per session.

CRITERION: Ninety-five percent (95%) correct responses over a four-day period.

DATA COLLECTION: After each trial, give a plus (+) for a correct response, and a minus (-) for a partial response shaped to completion, or a zero (0) when the resident makes no attempt and resists shaping or modelling.

GOAL: To make eye contact.

OBJECTIVE: To teach the resident to imitate actions modelled by the trainer.

MATERIALS: As required for each behavior and reinforcement.

SETTING: As required.

PROCEDURE

Using the behavior to be modelled for the resident, the trainer should say to the resident, "John/Jane, do this" and perform the action him or herself. Immediately the trainer should reinforce the resident with the appropriate reinforcers if he or she performs the desired action correctly. If the resident does not imitate the response, the trainer must physically assist the resident to perform the desired behavior (prompting). This process should be repeated until the resident correctly imitates without assistance 95% over a four day period and then repeat the procedure for the next task assigned. (See Note 2). The trainer should gradually fade his or her prompting assistance until the resident performs the response on his or her own. For example, the trainer may initially assist the resident to raise his or her left arm by taking the resident's hand and raising it for him or her. After several trials of this sort, the trainer should begin to gradually fade out assistance by raising the resident's arm only part way and shaping the completion of the response, i.e., the trainer should raise the resident's arm less and less high on each trial until he or she does it completely on his or her own. Use a similar procedure with other behaviors, i.e., help him or her a little less each time.

The resident resists physical assistance, the trainer should wait a short time and try again until even a partial response can be obtained without great resistance (for example, the resident's arm can at least be partially raised for the resident and reinforced).

In the beginning, edible and social reinforcement will be given immediately after each time the resident imitates to completion, reinforcement is given immediately after the trials (see Note 1) as the resident begins to respond consistently with a minimum amount of assistance. Consult with training supervisor and/or professional in charge to change the number of edible reinforcements given. Record the data on the sheet provided. Record a plus (+) mark if the resident imitates by himself when the trainer models and says, "John/Jane, do this", record a minus (-) sign if the resident partially imitates with the trainer giving physical assistance to complete the behavior, record zero (0) if the resident will not attempt to respond and resists assistance. Train each resident for five (5) minutes per session unless he or she becomes agitated and uncontrollable. In such cases, go on to another resident and return to that resident later.

Note 1: Since edible reinforcement will be given every trial at this point, all edibles must be broken into small pieces so that the resident does not get tired of them.

Note 2: If it is apparent that the resident is not learning to imitate a particular behavior, evaluate the resident in terms of physical disabilities, drugs given, etc. Consult with medical staff in this matter. This should have been done prior to the resident having been placed in this program and for that matter any training program. In some cases the "eye contact" procedures may have to be used in conjunction with the modelling procedure, i.e., before the command is given, the trainer must get the resident's attention.

CHAPTER TEN

SHAPING AND FADING PROCEDURES

Shaping and Fading Procedures for
25 Imitative Responses

Response	Shaping Procedure	Fading Procedure
1. Raise an arm	Lift at wrist	1. Less pressure at wrist 2. Backward to elbow 3. Finger touch at elbow
2. Stand up	Gesture and lift at shoulders	1. Lessen pressure at shoulder 2. Reduce gesture 3. Slight gesture
3. Sit on chair	Gesture and hands on shoulder, push downward	Same as above
4. Clap hands	Forced clap at wrist	1. Reduce pressure 2. Backward to elbow 3. Finger touch at elbow
5. Touch Head	Guided at wrist	Same as above
6. Touch mouth	Guided at wrist	Same as above

7. Pick up cup	Guided at wrist (Finger Closure if necessary)	1. Fade finger closure to wrist guidance 2. Reduce pressure 3. Backward to elbow
8. Touch table	Guided at wrist	1. Reduce pressure 2. Backward to elbow 3. Finger touch at elbow
9. Make a mark	Grasp fingers, close them around pencil	1. Fade finger closure to wrist assistance 2. Same as above (steps 1-3)
10. Touch wall	Grasp wrist and palm	1. Reduce pressure 2. Backward to elbow 3. Touch elbow
11. Touch floor	Grasp wrist and place other hand on shoulder, push downward	1. Reduce pressure on shoulder 2. Move wrist guidance to elbow 3. Finger touch to elbow
12. Arms outstretched	Grasp at wrist -pull toward you	1. Reduce pressure 2. Move wrists guidance to fingertips
13. Extend both arms away from sides	Grasp mid forearm, guide upwards and away from sides	1. Reduce guidance 2. Reduce upward guidance

		3. Finger touch to forearm
14. Clap thighs	Guide at wrists	1. Reduce pressure 2. Touch wrists
15. Touch knee	Guide at wrists	Same as above
16. Touch toes	Guide at wrists and place other hand on shoulder, push down-ward	1. Reduce pressure on shoulder 2. Reduce pressure on wrist 3. Finger touch to Wrist
17. Touch stomach	Guide at wrist	1. Reduce pressure 2. Move wrist guidance toward elbow 3. Finger touch to Elbow
18. Lift leg	Two hands under knee; lift	1. Reduce pressure
19. Smile	Index finger or thumbs at corners of mouth, Push outward	1. Reduce pressure 2. Finger touch at corners of mouth
20. Nod yes	Hands on chin and top of head, nod head	1. Reduce pressure of hand on head 2. Reduce pressure of hand on chin 3. Finger touch to Chin

21. Wave hello	Grasp wrist, move hand sideways while arm is near vertical	1. Reduce pressure 2. Backward to elbow 3. Finger touch to Elbow
22. Pick up ball	Grasp hand, guide it around ball	Same as above
23. Place arm thru Loop	Guide at wrist	Same as above
24. Jump up and down	Two hands on waist, T jumps up and down	1. T stops jumping 2. Reduce pressure 3. Finger touch to sides
25. Put ball in cup	Grasp hand; guide it around ball, open grip when ball is over cup	1. Reduce pressure 2. Backward to elbow 3. Finger touch to elbow

CHAPTER ELEVEN

COMMAND TRAINING, SIMPLE COMMANDS

OBJECTIVE: To teach the resident to follow simple verbal instructions.

MATERIALS: As required for each behavior.

SETTINGS: As required.

<u>PROCEDURE A</u>

Using behaviors which have previously been taught during imitation stage, the resident will be taught to follow simple verbal instructions. The trainer will give the command only once after he has gotten the attention (eye contact) of the resident by calling his or her name and/or by moving the reinforcer in front of the resident's face. The trainer may call the resident's name as many times as necessary to gain the resident's attention. The trainer may not proceed in giving the command until he or she has the attention of the resident. A single trial is defined as each time a command is given, i.e., "John/Jane, go to your room". If the resident makes the incorrect response, the trainer should immediately (within 3 seconds) physically assist the resident to perform the task requested, gradually decreasing physical assistance until the resident obeys command.

Reinforcement procedures and training time are the same as for imitation. If the resident resists shaping, the trainer should wait a short time and try again until the response can be obtained without great assistance.

TRAINING SESSION: Six (6) minutes per resident.

CRITERION: Ninety-Five (95) percent correct response rate over a four (4) day period.

NOTE: Beginning with the second command taught, the trainer should give five (5) random trials of previously learned commands in order to insure that the resident has learned to discriminate one command from another. At the end of the training, the resident should obey all commands when given by the trainer, in a random order.

COMMAND TRAINING, SIMPLE COMMANDS

OBJECTIVE: To teach Resident to follow simple verbal instructions.
MATERIALS: As required for each behavior.
SETTING: As required

R = RESIDENT
T = TRAINER

PROCEDURE B

Using behaviors which have previously been taught during the imitation stage, R will be taught to follow simple verbal instructions. T will give the command only once after he or she has gotten the attention (eye contact) of R by calling his or her name moving the reinforcer in front of R's face. T may call R's name as many times as necessary to gain R's attention. T may not proceed in giving the command until he has the attention of R. A single trial is defined as each correct response, T should immediately (within 3 seconds) physically assist R to perform the task requested, gradually decreasing physical assistance until R obeys without assistance.

Reinforcement procedures and training time are the same as for imitation. If R resists shaping, T should wait a short time and try again until the response can be obtained without great assistance.

TRAINING SESSION: Six (6) minutes per resident.

CRITERION: Ninety-Five (95%) percent correct response rate over a four (4) day period.

NOTE: Beginning with the second command taught, T should give five (5) random trials of previously learned command in order to insure that R has learned to discriminate one command from another. At the end of training, R should obey all commands when given by T in a random order.

PROCEDURE C

Procedure B consists of the same procedures carried out above but on a new set of commands not previously taught during the development of imitation.

BEHAVIORS PREVIOUSLY TAUGHT

Command	Shaping Procedure	Fading Procedure
1. John, stand up	Gesture and lift at the shoulders.	1. Lessen pressure at Shoulder 2. Reduce gesture 3. Slight gesture 4. No gesture
2. John, sit in the chair	Gesture and hands on the chair	1. Lessen pressure at shoulder, push downward 2. Reduce gesture 3. Slight gesture 4. No gesture
3. John, pick up the chair	Guided at wrist T grasps the back of R's hand & closes it around the cup	1. Fade finger closure 2. Reduce pressure 3. Backward to elbow
4. John, make a mark	Grasp fingers, close them around pencil	1. Fade finger closure to wrist guidance 2. Backward to elbow 3. Finger touch at elbow
5. John, touch your stomach	Guide at wrist	1. Reduce pressure 2. Move wrist guidance toward elbow 3. Finger touch to elbow

6. John, touch your knee	Guide at wrist	1. Reduce pressure 2. Touch wrist
7. John, nod yes	Hands on chin & top of head, nod head	1. Reduce pressure of hand on head 2. Reduce pressure of hand on chin 3. Touch chin
8. John, wave hello	Grasp wrist, move hand sideways while arm is vertical	1. Reduce pressure 2. Backward to elbow 3. Finger touch to elbow

NEW BEHAVIORS

Command	Shaping Procedure	Fading Procedure
1. John, go to the window	From behind gently push toward the window	1. Less pressure and only half the distance. 2. Only a touch on the back to start R
2. John, open the door	Grasp wrist & place hand On door knob, closing finger and turning hand	1.Fade finger closure and wrist assistance 2. Reduce pressure 3. Backward to Elbow
3. John, pick up the spoon	Guide wrist & finger closure if necessary	1. Fade finger closure & wrist assistance 2. Backward to elbow 3. Finger touch at Elbow
4. John, put the chair under the table	Guide at wrist	1. Reduce pressure 2. Backward to elbow 3. Finger touch at elbow
5. John, shake your head no	Hand on chin & on top of head, moving head horizontally	1. Reduce pressure of hand on head 2. Reduce pressure of hand on chin 3. Finger touch to chin

| 6. John, come here | Assistant behind R nudges R forward to T | 1. Less pressure 2. Slight touch on shoulder 3. Gesture by trainer |

The lesson plans and information included in this book are examples used successfully by the author during his professional career when the elderly were experiencing skill loss. This is especially true when working with those elderly residents with Alzheimer's dementia. However, these plans or examples are in no way intended to interfere with your own ideas and creativity as a caregiver. You should modify the lesson plans included in this book to meet an individual's specific needs, if the plans are too ambitious for the resident with whom you are working. Further, you may choose to develop your own plan of therapeutic intervention using your own creativity and imagination to address their skill loss.

In conclusion, existing behavioral procedures for the elderly, as well as those with dementia, are continually being revised in the light of new scientific evidence, and new procedures are being developed. The behavior change procedures defined in this book represent the current state of the behavior analysis literature. Periodic revisions will be necessary to incorporate new methods as scientific research and findings occur.

REFERENCES

Abbott RD, White LR, Ross GW, Masaki KH, Curb JD, Petrovitch H., (2004). Walking and Dementia in Physically Capable Elderly Men. JAMA. 292:1447-1453.

ADEAR Center, (2002). Reflections on Memories Lost: Stories of Early Alzheimer's Disease With Expert Commentary on Symptoms, Diagnosis and Treatment from Dr. John C. Morris. Silver Springs, Md: ADEAR Center.

Aevarsson O, Skoog I, (1996). A Population-based Study on the Incidence of Dementia Disorders Between 85 and 88 Years of Age. J Am Geriatr Soc. 44: 1455-1460.

Alzheimer Caregiver's Handbook, (2003). Alzheimer's Foundation of the South Mississippi Division. Gulfport, MS.

American Psychiatric Association, (1995). Diagnostic and Statistical Manual of Mental Disorders, Revised Fourth Edition. Washington, DC: American Psychiatric Association.

American Psychiatric Association, (1997). Practice Guideline for The Treatment of Patients With Alzheimer's Disease And Other Dementias of Late Life. Am J Psychiatry: 154 (suppl 5): 1-39.

Aronson MK, Ooi WL, Geva DL, Masur D, Blau A, Friehman W., (1991). Dementia, Age-Dependant Incidence, Prevalence, and Mortality in the Old Old. Arch Intern Med. 151:989-992.

Azrin NH and Foxx RM., (1971). A Rapid Method of Toilet Training the Institutionalized Retarded. Journal of Applied Behavior Analysis. 4:89-99.

Bennett DA., (2004). Mild Cognitive Impairment. Clin Geriatr Med. 20:15-25.

Benson RR, Guttmann CR, Wei X, et al., (2002). Older People With Impaired Mobility Have Specific Loci of Periventricular Abnormality on MRI. Neurology. 58:48-55.

Bolla KI, Lindgren KN, Bonaccorsy C, Bleecker ML., (1991). Memory Complaints in Older Adults. Fact or Fiction? Arch Neurol. 48:61-64

Bookheimer SY, Strojwas MH, Cohen MS, et al., (2000). Patterns of Brain Activation in People at Risk for Alzheimer's Disease. N Engl J Med. 343: 450-456.

Bowirrat A, Treves TA, Friendland RP, Korczyn AD, (2001). Prevalance of Alzheimer's Type Dementia in an Elderly Arab Population. Eur J Neurol. 8:119-123.

Bullock R, Hammond G., (2003). Realistic Expectations: The Management of Severe Alzheimer's Disease. Alzheimer Dis Assoc Disord. 17 (suppl 3): S80-S85.

Chan DC, Kasper JD, Black BS, Rabins PV., (2003). Prevalence and Correlates of Behavioral and Psychiatric Symptoms in Community-dwelling Elders with Dementia or Mild Cognitive Impairment: The Memory and Medical Care Study. Int J Geriatr Psychiatry. 18: 174-182.

Clarfield AM. (2003). The Decreasing Prevalence of Reversible Dementias: An Updated Meta-Analysis. Arch Intern Med. 163:2219-2229.

Covinsky KE, Newcomer R, Fox P, et al., (2003). Patient and Caregiver Characteristics Associated With Depression in Caregivers of Patients With Dementia. J Gen Intern Med. 18:1006-1014.

Craig D, Hart DJ, McCool K, McIllroy SP, Passmore AP., (2004). Apolipo-protein E e4 Allele Influences Aggressive Behavior in Alzheimer's Disease. J Neurol Neurosurg Psychiatry. 75:1327-1330.

Doghcamji PP., (2001). Detection of Insomnia in Primary Care. J of Clinical Psychiatry. Vol. 62, Suppl. 10.

Doka K., (2001). Challenging the Paradigm; New Understanding of Grief. The College of New Rochelle, New York.

Foxx RM and Azrin NH., (1976). Toilet Training the Retarded.

Gray KF, (2004). Managing Agitation and Difficult Behavior in Dementia. Clin Geriatr Med, 20: 69-82.

Green RC, (2005), Diagnosis and Management of Alzheimer's Disease and Other Dementias. Professional Communications, Inc., Caddo, OK.

Griffith HR, Belue K, Sicola A., et al., (2003). Impaired Financial Abilities in Mild Cognitive Impairment: A Direct Assessment Approach. Neurology 60: 449-457.

Grundman J, Peterson RC, Ferris, SH, et al., (2004). Alzheimer's Disease Cooperative Study. Mild Cognitive Impairment Can Be Distinguished From

Alzheimer's Disease and Normal Aging For Clinical Trials. Arch Neurol 61: 59-66.

Hall VR., (1971). Managing Behavior. Part 1. Behavior Modification: The Measurement of Behavior. H. and H. Enterprises, Lawrence, KS.

Hall VR., (1971). Managing Behavior. Part II. Behavior Modification: Basic Principles. H. and H. Enterprises, Lawrence, KS.

Hall VR., (1971). Managing Behavior. Part III. Part III. Behavior Modification: Applications in School and Home. H. and H. Enterprises, Lawrence, KS.

Hirschman KB, James BD, Joyce, CM., et al., (2004). Do Alzheimer's Disease Patients Want To Participate in an AD Treatment Decision and Will Their Family Let Them? Neurobiol Aging 25:21.

Hurley AC, Volicer, L., (2002). Alzheimer's Disease: "It's Okay, Mama, If You Want To Go, It's Okay". JAMA 28.8:2324-2331.

Karlawish JH, Bonnia RJ, Appelbaum, PS, et al., (2004). Addressing the Ethical, Legal, and Social Issues Raised by Voting by Persons with Dementia. JAMA. 292:1345-1350.

Kawas CH, Corrada MM, Brookmeyer R., et al., (2003). Visual Memory Predicts Alzheimer's Disease Move Then a Decade Before Diagnosis. Neurology. 60:1689-1693.

Laughren T., (2000). Regulatory Issues on Behavioral and Psychological Symptoms of Dementia in the United States. International Psychogeriatrics, Vol. 12, Suppl. 1.

Linford MD, Hipsher LW, Silikovitz RG, (1972). Systematic Instruction for Retarded Children. The Interstate Printers & Publishers, Inc.

Maurar TA., (2002). Alzheimer's Care; Combining High-Tech with High-Touch. Responses to an Aging Florida. Atlanta, GA.

McShane R., (2000). What Are the Symptoms of Behavioral and Psychological Symptoms of Dementia? International Psychogeriatrics, Vol. 12, Suppl. 1.

Migiacclo JN., (2002). Advanced Monitoring Systems Provide Clues to Resident Challenges, Enabling Staff to Provide Better Care. Assisted Living Today, Vol. 9, No. 5. New York.

Ramage JW., (2006). Creating Therapeutic Activity Plans in Long Term Care Facilities: The Basic Principles. Authorhouse, Bloomington, IN.

Schulz R, Mendelsohn AB, Haley WE, et al., (2003). Resources for Enhancing Alzheimer's Caregiver Health Investigators. End of Life Care and the Effects of Bereavement on Family Caregivers of Persons with Dementia. New England Journal of Medicine. 349:1936-1942.

Skinner BF., (1953). Science and Human Behavior. MacMillan Co., New York.

Small SQ., (2001). Age Related Memory Decline. Current concepts and Future Directions. Arch Neurol., Vol. 58.

Ten I, Gibbons IE, McCurry SM., et al., (2002). Exercise Plus Behavioral Management in Patients with Alzheimer's Disease: A Randomized Controlled Trial. JAMA, 290: 2015-2022.

Teri L, Logsclon RG, McCurry SM., (2002). Nonpharmacologic Treatment of Behavioral Disturbance in Dementia. Med Clin North Am 86: 641-656.

Volicer I, Hurley AC., (2003). Management of Behavioral Symptoms in Progressive Degenerative Dementias. J Gerontology and Biological Science, Medical Science. 58: M837-M845.

Weintraub S., (2000). Neuropsychological Assessment of Mental State in Mesulam M-M, ed. Principles of Cognitive and Behavioral Neurology. 2nd ed. Oxford University Press, New York.

Weuve J, Kang JH, Manson JE, Bretaler MM, Ware JH, Grodstein F., (2004). Physical Activity, Including Walking, and Cognitive Function in Older Women. JAMA 292: 1454-1461.

Wild K, Catrell V., (2003). Identifying Driving Impairment in Alzheimer's Disease: A Comparison of Self and Observer Reports Versus Driving Evaluation. Alzheimer Dis. Assoc. 17: 27-34.

Wimo A, Winbald B, Aguero-Tones, Von Suauss B., (2003). The Magnitude of Dementia Occurrence in the World. Alzheimer's Dis Assoc Disord. 17:63-67.

Wilson RS, Beckett LA., et al., (2003). Individual Dofferences in Rates of Change in Cognitive Abilities of Older Persons. Psychology of Aging 17: 179-193.

Wilson RD, Mendes, De Leon CF, Barnes LL., et al., (2002). Participation in Cognitively Stimulating Activities and Risk of Incident Alzheimer's Disease. JAMA 287: 742-748.

Zeisel J, Silverstein NM, Hyde J, Levkoff S, Lawton MP, Holmes W., (2003). Environmental Correlates in Behavioral Health Outcomes in Alzheimer's Special Care Units. Gerontologist 43: 697-711.

Zubenko GA., (2000). Neurobiology of Major Depression in Alzheimer's Disease. International Psychiatrics. Vol 12, Suppl. 1.

ABOUT THE AUTHOR

Dr. Ramage's career spans over forty years in the Field of Human Services. He holds graduate degrees in both Clinical Social Work and Behavioral Psychology, followed by post graduate training in behavior modification, behavior and cognitive therapy. He is a Diplomate in Clinical Social Work, a Fellow and Diplomate in Medical Psychotherapy, and is an Activity Consultant Certified with the National Certification Council for Activity Professionals. He is listed in Who's Who in the American Academy of Human Services and in Who's Who Among Service Professionals. Dr. Ramage has practiced in both the public and private sectors in mental health and nursing home industry. During his career, he has worked as a clinician, educator, administrator, manager, consultant, and is the author of numerous professional articles and books.

He presently serves on the Staff of The Bibb Medical Center in Centreville, Alabama, a large medical, skilled nursing home, retirement village, and human services complex. Dr. Ramage has extensive professional experience with programs serving older persons and has developed policy intervention strategies for practitioners, administrators, educators and researchers in the area of gerontology. He is best known for administering a home mental health component and the development of intergenerational practice models. Dr. Ramage resides in Northport, AL with his wife, Margaret, where he maintains a private practice.

He can be contacted regarding consultation, workshops, and conferences, by e-mail: ramagejamesphd@earthlink.net.